THE WISE OLD MAN

THE WISE OLD MAN

Healing through Inner Images

Pieter Middelkoop

Translated by Adrienne Dixon
Foreword by Robert Bosnak

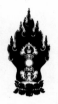

SHAMBHALA
Boston & Shaftesbury
1989

Shambhala Publications, Inc.
Horticultural Hall
300 Massachusetts Avenue
Boston, Massachusetts 02115

9 8 7 6 5 4 3 2 1

First Edition
Printed in the United States of America on acid-free paper

Library of Congress Cataloging-in-Publication Data

Middelkoop, Pieter, 1929–
    The wise old man.

    Translation of: Oude wijze man.
    Bibliography: p.
    1. Imagination—Therapeutic use.   2. Imagery (Psychology)—
Therapeutic use.   3. Psychotherapy.
I. Title.
RC489.F35M5313   1989   616.89′14   89-46233

CONTENTS

FOREWORD

You are about to enter a therapy of the imagination through tales of interaction between our conscious selves and the archaic imagination, the birthplace of all images. Psychotherapist Pieter Middelkoop follows closely the path described by Jung, convinced that there is an unconscious core of Self, which, like a distant and forever invisible command force in interior space, steers consciousness through life. What was from ancient times called the guiding spirit is often envisioned and interiorly seen as a Wise Old Man, an archaic character of collective soul that lives buried deeply in everyone. The contact we have to this archetypal undercurrent—this inner therapist, as Middelkoop calls it—is through the imagination.

Jung discovered a therapy of the imagination. He called it active imagination to differentiate it from passive reverie. Faced with a direct personal experience of spontaneous immersion in the world of unconscious images, Jung let himself drop into his imagination and interacted with the personages he met in this dreamlike reality, in the same way one interacts with other real creatures. Through this therapy of self, Jung found his own inner sense of direction, his guiding spirit, imagined as the Wise Old Man.

Middelkoop will make you acquainted with the developments that the primordial image world and human consciousness undergo while interacting with each other. He shows how the imagination can torment us, as well as loosen us from the fixated bondages we have to the same old ruts, thus opening up new vistas to lives lived in a world that has become too small.

Middlekoop tells true stories about the life of people he sees in therapy, where he uses active imagination as the primary form of treatment. Staying close to actual cases, he probes each imaginer's experiences, encouraging him or her to communicate with the fairy-tale-like world of archaic consciousness. And as we follow the adventures of others, Middelkoop leads us all to the men, women, and other creatures that populate the deep.

In Pieter Middelkoop's book we learn the art of active imagination by demonstration. This gives the necessary body to practical guidelines given at the conclusion of the text. It will be a guide to anyone who wants to practice active imagination, whether as a therapist of others, of self, or both.

Robert Bosnak

THE WISE OLD MAN

INTRODUCTION

Few of us are aware that it is in principle possible to live alternately in two worlds: an inner world and an outer world. We are accustomed to living only in the outer world and that is the focus of our lives. We have made ourselves as familiar with this world as it is possible to be, and our parents and teachers have done their utmost to explain to us how this world is put together and how one can best survive in it.

However, there is also an inner world, although in modern times we have to some degree lost sight of it. That world still exists, and under certain circumstances it is possible for us to get in touch with it again. This happens in various forms of psychotherapy, for instance in imagination therapy. That is what this book is about. It contains the accounts of several people who entered this inner world of the imagination, in an attempt to tackle and as far as possible overcome their psychological problems.

When we speak of the world of the imagination, this may give rise to a number of superficial misunderstandings. The word *imagination* has acquired a particular association that does not do justice to the concept. For instance, we might be under the illusion that we can imagine anything we like in this inner world of ours. But that is not the case. The inner world conforms only partly to our wishes, desires and intentions. For the rest, what is conjured up before us is likely to surprise us, because we would never consciously have thought of such a world ourselves. Its images rise up from the unconscious areas of our personality, and we can influence them only to some extent. A second kind of misunderstanding may arise, namely that we have 'only imagined' a particular thing. Such a remark would suggest that we have made a mistake and that we thought we observed something which in fact was not really there at all. In a sense this is true, we have imagined something and we have done so in our inner world, while we thought, in error, that we were dealing with something in the outer world. A wrong assessment of this kind demonstrates clearly that we must keep the inner and outer worlds well separated from each other.

In order to escape such misunderstandings, we have chosen the term *imaginal world* and we will use the term *imagination* in a particular sense: a description of an experience in this imaginal world. These imaginations have a great deal to do with our life as it is and with the way in which we live. We will meet our joys and our sorrows there, but also our anxieties and, for example, the difficulties we have in our relationships with other people. All these things are expressed in visible, moving images and we are in the midst of these images. We are fully alert to what is going on, so that you might say you are dreaming while you are awake. You are in the realm of your imagination, in your imaginal inner world.

This is a world in which we can experience all manner of things and in which we can encounter our problems in an entirely new situation, with the possibility of solving them. The imaginal world is preeminently a world which challenges us to conquer our difficulties. Sometimes it does so by setting us specific tasks, at other moments by putting various things before us. As a result we find ourselves in a fairy-tale-like happening that appears to have been organized from a central point. We shall call this point the core of the Self. This is not to be thought of as an abstract point, for our core presents itself in a personified form. It is a person, with whom we can have contact and who in turn develops initiatives with regard to us or who features in the background as a guiding hand when other figures are active in the dramatic situation. Very probably this core figure is present right from the start of any imagination, as a kind of film director, but usually shows itself only much later, when all the preparatory work has been done.

A person who enters the imaginal world will at first probably not quite know what to do with the things he or she sees there.

The director's hand is often not very readily perceived in the early stages and it may be difficult to recognize the positive nature of the imaginal situation. The same may also happen to you, the reader, when, somewhat unprepared, you are suddenly confronted with the strange events that take place. You will therefore do well to bear the same points in mind as the imaginator. You must continually ask yourself: "What does the content of this imagination situation have to do with my daily existence? To what can I relate these events? What do I recognize in them? What might the film director have in mind for me?" And, especially if the experience does not promise to be very pleasant, "What is the meaning of the situation in which I find myself?"

This last question, about the meaning of the imaginations, is extremely important. We have become too accustomed to the idea that our unconscious produces mostly frightening images, and it is often hard to accept the notion that the purpose of such images can nevertheless be positive. All the same, the imagination therapy that I shall be describing is based upon the knowledge that imaginations, once they are under way, always aim, to a greater or lesser degree, to exercise a favorable influence on our life. This is true even when the imagination is unpleasant.

The inner images therefore form the first starting point of the therapy, and the first place we try to come to terms with our problems is in the experience of the imagination itself. In the conversations both before and after an imagination we can search for links with our daily life. The imaginal world creates a field of force in which certain developments become possible while everything else becomes much more difficult, which means that we are able to tap new sources in ourselves.

How exactly imaginations come about will be described more fully in Chapter 4. For the moment we are mostly interested in the question of how we can work with them therapeutically, and for this reason I give a step by step account of some therapies for you, the reader, to follow.

Imaginations are in the first place intended to give us an insight into the unconscious forces that play a part in our lives.

Why is it, we ask ourselves, that certain things which we attempt in our lives go wrong time and again, for no reason that we can understand? We may react by getting angry, or by waiting resignedly until things get better. We may look to other people in the hope that they will find a solution for us. Whatever our response, it remains a gamble, because we do not really know what is going on. Something incomprehensible is taking place inside us; we seem unable to get a clear view of it and we keep getting stuck in the same blind alley. Imaginations can provide us with the key to the hidden reason we fail time and time again in our aspirations, and are perhaps bound to fail because we are seeking the solution in the wrong direction. At times the images present us with a situation that seems to be a clear diagnosis of the difficulties in which we find ourselves. The very first imagination described in this book, the one titled "The Dwarf and the Strawberry Plant," is an obvious example of this.

The second starting point for therapy can be found in the positive forces that are active in our unconscious. It is often possible to create more room for these forces. Our aim must therefore be to track them down, and find out why they have so far been so relatively ineffective and what can be done to improve their performance. Often imaginators may be quite unaware that such positive unconscious forces exist. They believe that there is nothing but woe and misery in their inner world, and they will therefore be inclined not to dig too deeply, because this would only create further distress. Since they have no contact at all with these internal forces they assume that they do not exist.

When I speak of 'forces' in this context, I do not mean anything abstract. In the imaginations these forces appear as persons or as animals, and sometimes as wonderfully strange beings quite unlike any we have ever encountered in our ordinary world.

It is possible to make contact with these figures, and to get to know the forces they represent. However, getting to know these forces does not necessarily lead to an immediately favorable appreciation. The encounter can also lead to the thought "which of us two is mad?" Sometimes the inner figures show us in no uncertain terms that we have gotten hold of the wrong end of the stick. However, if we are prepared to take a hint, we will realize that things can begin to move forward again in our life, and that a helping hand is being extended to us. Another of our initial assumptions is, therefore, that neither the imaginator nor any figure in the imaginal world is mad. What matters is that they will meet and understand each other. As we shall see later, the imaginal figures speak a language all of their own, and it will be necessary to learn that language, as a means of communication. Once this means of communication has been found, we can get started. The journey has then really begun and, if you wish, it can turn out to be a voyage of adventure.

Imaginations can therefore be regarded as voyages through an inner world of images. In this book several sequences of imaginations are described and explained. They originate with different people and must therefore also be seen against different backgrounds. In the explanatory comments, I give brief outlines of these various backgrounds so that the reader will be able to empathize with the psychological reality represented in the imaginations of the person concerned. The sequences of imaginations form the basis of the first three chapters of the book. In each chapter the therapy of one person is shown in images. I have deliberately chosen therapies of very different kinds.

Chapter 1 describes the process by which the ego, the person himself, and the unknown forces in the imaginal world—we might also say "the unconscious"—at first follow very divergent courses, but eventually move together in the same direction.

In Chapter 2 a process is shown in which there is a conflict between different unconscious forces in the imaginal world, to which the ego initially seems to be a complete outsider. Only gradually does the ego begin to take part in what is going on, and this eventually brings about an integration within the person as a whole.

Chapter 3 tackles problems that are not strictly personal. After all, the difficulties we have to cope with do not always concern ourselves alone. Sometimes we share them with large numbers of other people in the same cultural environment as ourselves. For example, there are the problems of violence in our society, and of discrimination against the feminine in our culture (which must not be equated with discrimination against women, although the two are related). In order to allow people to see and empathize with what happens in an imagination, I had to find participants who were willing not only to make their imaginations public but also to divulge a certain amount of information about their personal lives. Fortunately there was such willingness, and I am most grateful to the people concerned, and also to those who made fragments of their imaginations available, which made it possible to explain various points in Chapter 4.

The information that was made available can be found partly in the commentaries and partly in the utterances of the imaginators themselves. The commentaries are in every case addressed to the imaginator. This enables you, the reader, to form an idea of the personal atmosphere in which I work with my clients. The interpretations incorporated in these chapters were often arrived at during conversations over a span of time. Their position in this book is not always the same as the position in which they were expressed in reality. Some of the observations have existed for long periods only in the mind of the accompanist/therapist.

Finally, Chapter 4 contains a number of technical and theoretical points, however tentative. I tried to find connections with what others have previously found in their investigations. In particular, I have paid attention to a description of various phenomena that commonly occur in the imaginal worlds of many people.

IF WE NOW return to the world of the inner imaginations, we can say that this world is partly known to the imaginator, that is to say, it is known to him in so far as it contains images that are derived from his daily reality and that appear to him by means of some kind of visual memory. The rest, however, consists of unfamiliar images, which do not originate directly with the imaginator's experience in the external world. They can be compared with dream images, which rise up from the unconscious.

The traveler in this inner world of images can decide for himself which course he wishes to take. The journey can be made on foot or by some other form of transport. There are roads and crossroads, and at every turn the traveler will have to ask himself: "Shall I go left, right, or straight ahead? Can I see something that appeals to me or am I repelled by anything?"

He will also meet opposition. The images and representations exercise their influence on him, and besides, there are phenomena in the inner world that are unknown in the world outside. Certain laws apply there that are of an entirely different nature from any that apply elsewhere.

It is not actually necessary to know these phenomena and laws in advance. As soon as you enter an imagination, you must begin to learn. It is a special kind of learning, which concentrates on sensibility and empathy. You cannot really prepare yourself in advance for what is going to happen. You will find out in due course what is being asked of you; it will gradually become clear.

You can begin the journey into your inner self by closing yourself off from the outside world for a while, concentrating instead on the inner world of images. To most people this immediately suggests a world of visual images, but it does not have to be that. Some people simply 'feel' where they are and yet can describe in detail what it all looks like. Others inhabit mostly a world of sound, and can quite easily embark on lengthy conversations with people they are unable, or hardly able, to see.

Once you have some idea of where you are, the actual journey can begin. First of all you try to establish your own position in the imaginal world. Are you perhaps watching from a hilltop or are you walking along a country lane picking flowers? Are you hovering in the air or are you under water?

You might be some place where normally, in the external world, it would be impossible for you to be. Here, in the inner world, such things are possible. Here you can float endlessly above a landscape, and eventually decide to make a landing, at any point that you choose. You can also walk under water while continuing to breathe normally. There again, you can move in any direction, and you may encounter all sorts of beings that live under the water.

One of the most striking features of this inner world is the fact that in certain cases it is not the traveler who decides where the journey will lead but some other force. Of course, this confronts us with a problem, for what should we imagine "some other force" to be? Current opinion would expect action only from the side of the ego, the traveler himself. But this is not the case here; there is a second force at work.

In order to give our thoughts about these matters some kind of anchorage, we will link them to the ideas of Carl Gustav Jung.[1] In his personality model he takes two basic concepts as his starting point: the ego and the Self. Of these two, the Self is the more comprehensive concept. It applies to the totality of the human personality, and according to Jung's way of thinking it encompasses both the unconscious and the conscious areas of the person. The conscious part is rather like an island surrounded by water, the water being the unconscious part, which is far, far larger than the conscious part.

As we have said earlier, the ego rules in the conscious part of the personality. Within the Self, Jung presupposes a center[2] in which the forces of the unconscious are organized. This center we have called the *core of the Self*.

When this core of the Self becomes active, the inner images increasingly begin to show a distinct tendency to work toward a specific aim. This aim is pursued jointly by the ego and the core of the Self. The actions of the core become visible in the different imaginal figures that cross your path. One of these may be an animal, which to your surprise asks you a question, such as where you are going and what you want to do there. Maybe it will tell you that it would be better for you to take a different direction. As the imagination progresses, the actions of the core will be controlled more and more by one single being, who takes charge of the proceedings. We see, then, that the images in the inner world of the Self are partly realistic. However, there are also surrealist images, as well as images from the realm of myths, fairytales, and fables. This is one of the reasons why one can perhaps speak of a fairy-tale or fabulous Self. Another reason is the fact that the Self appears to know what is good and what is bad for human life and that, moreover, it is capable of exercising a strong favorable influence on our life. The imaginations in this book demonstrate this unconscious knowledge and its effects sufficiently clearly for you to gain an impression of them.

Although we use the word *fabulous* here to indicate the guiding action of the core of the Self, this does not mean that we now have a solution to all our problems. Alas, we do not. In Chapter 4 we shall come back to this point. At any rate, the imaginations described in this book show that there are good opportunities for further growth and a chance to settle with the past. The imaginations came about during weekly therapy sessions, each lasting about one hour. Part of that time, about fifteen to twenty minutes, is spent in an imagination. The therapist is present during this time and the imaginator relates what he or she experiences and undertakes during the journey in the inner world. The experiences are noted down verbatim, and this is how they have been presented in this book. Everything has been left as authentic as possible. Only here and there some passages have been polished slightly in order to make them more readable, but they have not been altered in any material way or embellished to give them literary elegance. The information given by the imaginator is usually fairly brief and terse, which is not surprising when we consider how many different tasks someone has to perform on one of these journeys. The world which is being entered is a totally unfamiliar one, and the imaginator has to absorb new impressions all the time, and make decisions practically every minute.

In addition, there is someone present beside the imaginator—the accompanist/therapist, who puts in a word from time to time and poses questions or asks his or her attention for something or other. It is therefore an extremely complicated process, which is occasionally charged with emotion. The total reality of such an event cannot possibly be written down on paper, but I have tried my best to do so.

The imaginations recorded here are only a small selection from a large number. I have chosen them with the aim of demonstrating the inner direction of the sequence. Although it seems as if something different is happening all the time, it gradually becomes possible to discern a certain line in it. The main task for the accompanist is to try and discover the course of the process and to support it.

The question is therefore always: What is the core of the Self aiming for? And how does the ego respond to this? What is the result of the interaction between the two?

Following this, there is a second question: What would be a sensible contribution from outside? In the imaginations, the Self speaks a language of its own. It is the language of images, metaphors, symbols, and rituals. We have to find a way to link up with this. Life in the imaginal world can be fully lived in every respect. It is not a visual world only: you can also taste what there is to eat and smell whatever there is to be smelled. And you can exchange thoughts and have conversations.

As I have already said, many kinds of beings occur in this world, some of whom may be figures from fairy tales and myths. The gods often put in an appearance and can burst in upon us at any time, even if we have long ceased to believe in them. You can refuse to make contact with the figures that appear before you, but this is not easy, especially in the case of mythological and divine beings, because they are often very impressive.

We speak of "divine beings" in order to distinguish between them and the God we may presume to exist outside ourselves. The connection between the divine beings within us and the God who stands behind everything is emphatically suggested in the images. This happens, for instance, in the case of the figure called Eternal in Chapter 2. In other examples, the connection with God is explicitly stated by the divine figures themselves.

IN ORDER TO form an idea of what exactly the imaginations stand for, we need some information about the daily lives of the imaginators. Without this, their stories remain simply stories, with a bit of packaged wisdom here and there. But we have to look at them differently. The images are related to the way in which the imaginators live and with the problems they encounter in their lives. The stories are therefore not simply stories but interpretations of the way in which the ego gets on with the Self, or doesn't, as the case may be.

There are no fixed guidelines for the way in which this interplay should be enacted, and this is why entering upon an imagination is a true, real-life adventure. The ego strives for something but so does the Self, and the ego may be confronted with difficult tasks. This goes on until the ego has sufficiently gained in strength or else has descended from its pedestal in order to find a mode of life that enables it to live in constructive harmony with the Self.

To the extent that symbols occur in imaginations, it is not always necessary to understand them. In some cases understanding may even be a hindrance. Symbols do not only serve to reveal something; they can also, where necessary, conceal.

One might say that the unconscious part of the Self is not always prepared to state explicitly what it is doing. We need a certain degree of respect in our dealings with it.[3] At certain moments the Self is emphatically silent. Symbols, then, do not always need to be interpreted. They simply carry out their task, which is that of exercising influence, and this task can still be performed even when you do not understand the symbolism. In these circumstances it is important to allow them to exercise their influence on oneself and, if possible, to find out what effect they are having.

There are often moments at which the "director" of the imagination seems to know where you are, what you have understood and what you haven't. The images are then adapted to this situation, and new ones will arise to make further development possible, until the moment has arrived in which the message can be stated explicitly. Often you will be told, when asking a question to which you would, at that moment, not understand the answer: "That will come later, it isn't the right time for that yet."

Of course, this is all very mysterious. When we engage ourselves in the inner world, mystery returns to our lives. This often happens right at the beginning, when, during the first meeting with a core figure, whom you have never met before, you are told: "I have been waiting for you. It's taken you so long! I am glad you have come."

I could attempt to explain much more, but at this stage it is inevitable that there will be some things that are hard to understand. No doubt far more study is needed to clear up numerous mysteries.

In my efforts to put into words what I thought I understood, and to do so as clearly as possible, I have been greatly assisted by J. M. C. van der Goes, who was willing to read this book and criticize it on the basis of his experience in psychiatric practice. I have made grateful use of your criticism, Jan, even if at times I appeared to be stubborn. Many thanks.

1–SETTLING ACCOUNTS WITH THE PAST

The Dwarf and the Strawberry Plant

It looks like a toadstool. But I can see a very thin stalk. It is a strawberry, at the top of a very thin little stalk. There is also a dwarf, busy with a watering can.

Behind the dwarf someone is raking the ground, and digging a hole. It is a witch. The stalk becomes thicker and thicker and then the strawberry falls on the ground. The witch has been waiting for this, and she also has designs on the dwarf. She wants to rake everything into a heap. I feel I am that dwarf.

I don't quite know what to think of all this. The next thing I see is a skeleton lying on the ground. This is very odd, because it is still wearing boots. Then the skeleton changes. It looks as though it is becoming a person again. The person sits up. It is a medieval knight, drawing his sword. He lashes out left and right. He attacks the witch. He hacks her to pieces completely. I feel angry too.

There is someone else near by. I can't see him very well. To judge by his clothes I would say he is probably a gardener. I also feel that he is a father. But I cannot see his head. Let me try, though. It is all rather scary. He has very peculiar eyes. Big rolling eyes. His whole head is scary. It is a monstrous sort of head. I am frightened of him.

Now I see a luminous figure in the sky. It is the Virgin Mary. I cannot hold on to her image. Something like a spinning top comes between us. And a crocodile with wide open mouth. A little boy is playing with the spinning top. That is me. Now the crocodile whirls around like a train. The spinning top topples over.

In the distance I see two pairs of children's legs dangling over the edge of a canal. I suppose they must be fishing. I go up to them. One of them is a girl. I try to get closer and make contact with her. When I am very close she changes into a dove. The dove flies away, swerves in a large curve and comes back again. Now it is no longer a dove, it has become a bird of prey, which looks very dangerous. The bird flies away again. Now it has become a dove once more. It describes another large curve and then it changes into a bird of prey again. And then into a dove again.

I stop doing this.

A First Analysis

We had just been talking about those constant, never-ending feelings of anxiety. You are thirty-three years old now and there is a lot of anger inside you. You never seem to manage to live happily as a man on your own. Unlike most other people, you have no family. Instead, you usually live alone, occasionally sharing with a friend, but it has never come to anything, as though it were impossible to have a good relationship with a man of your own age. On the other hand, you are always assailed by feelings of anxiety whenever you meet much younger boys with whom you fall in love and who arouse strong feelings in you. It can only lead to a lot of misery, so you think.

And now you don't even dare go out into the street anymore to buy the things that might give you a little pleasure. Never a cream cake any more, or a piece of sausage. And better put off having the car repaired, so you are forced to go out on foot after all, with your belly full of fear. Off to the baker's store, but when you get there you are unable to utter a word when the woman asks you what you want, so you run home again without any cakes. So then you are back in the place where the walls stare at you and your fear grips you by the throat.

You arrive at the first therapy session and when you have given an acount of all these things that torment you, you are asked to close your eyes for a while and look at the images that live inside you. What you then see is the story of the dwarf and the strawberry plant, as it has been recorded here. It is not a very cheering story. On the contrary, it makes you feel wretched. Luckily, there have been better images since then. After a time you were able to say, "After unpleasant images I feel very wretched. When they are nice, I feel moved, and that makes me feel good."

At first you found it difficult to believe in the images, and from time to time you thought they were only making you feel worse. It was necessary to talk about them often and by doing so to discover that at the end of unpleasant imaginations about death and unhappiness there was always something hopeful as well, something that pointed to a new beginning. Yes, in the early days the images were not cheerful. You had to look very hard to find anything hopeful in them. And yet even the very first imaginations already contained signs of hope, even though these were often well hidden. This is very realistic, because real life is exactly the same: a few glimmers of light here and there while the rest is dark. Let us therefore have a closer look at the story.

To begin with, there is a strawberry plant on a thin stalk. No good will ever come of that, you might say. But things don't go wrong at once. There is a dwarf, who waters the plant. You can feel empathy with that. The stalk becomes thicker, and this is encouraging. It even seems as if the fruit is about to ripen and drop off. Up to that point there is hope. But then there is that witch with her rake, and soon enough her destructive intentions become clear. She wants to get at the strawberry plant and also at the dwarf. She digs a hole for them both. The dwarf can see the danger, but there is little he can do to defend himself. You, the imaginator, recognize your own situation in the scene. You have little defense against the course of events. You are small and the witch is big. In this situation you look around to see if any help can be expected. There does not seem much hope. You see a skeleton lying on the ground, which is in itself reason for further anxiety. Here it appears, however, that in the language of the imaginal world dead does not mean dead.[1] Following your surprise that the skeleton is still wearing its boots, you notice that it is beginning to show life. Gradually, a complete knight comes into being. He turns out to be capable of defeating the witch. What can this mean? You, as imaginator, have immediately joined ranks with the dwarf, but there is something appealing about the knight too. They are both parts of yourself. This means that you have the possibility of being a knight. This does not solve all your problems at once, but all the same there must be something brave in you which is willing to fight evil.

When you look around a bit more, you see the gardener with his monstrous head. At first he reminds you of a father figure, but the head with the rolling eyes makes you lose all confidence in him.

This encounter with the gardener and the witch awakens memories of the past in you. You remember that even as a child you were very timid and had little confidence in your own parents. It is this fearfulness that has become visible in these two frightening figures. This is not pleasant for you, but at least you can do something about it now. For the moment the two figures make you feel afraid, but they need not continue to do so. Certainly not now that you have joined ranks with the knight. The more you fight on his side, the more you will notice that the frightening figures disappear from the scene. And when they do, you will probably be able to get on better with your real parents. At this moment, however, you have to face up to the fact that these figures form part of yourself, and that makes the reality of every day into a grim business.

When we look more closely at the images, we see that there is also a child playing with a spinning top. The Virgin Mary watches, but she is not alone. There is a crocodile too. Its wide open mouth is enough to terrify the child. The top stops spinning. The child's play has been spoilt utterly.

The images that follow next are still part of the child's world, however. Your attention is drawn to two pairs of children's legs dangling over the edge of a canal. You feel attracted toward those children and you go up to them. When you get closer it seems that your preference is for the little girl. This makes me think. What can be going on? You have told me you don't get on with girls and that you have therefore focused your whole life on boys and men. So why do you now choose a girl? For the moment this is not quite clear and if I were to ask you, you would probably not know the answer. The only thing that can be said with certainty is that the girl changes into a dove. In other words, the encounter is not successful, but the dove holds out a promise. However, the bird returns from its flight as a bird of prey, and this is a frightening factor. Clearly there is a certain ambivalence in you: you are hoping to receive something from this encounter and yet at the same time you are afraid of it.

Earlier on we briefly mentioned the strawberry plant, but we have not gone into this very closely. The girl was tricky enough, but the image of the plant is even more difficult. In the books it says that this stands for the sweet fruit of marriage, for the life together with wife and children.[2] Very deep down inside you there must therefore be a longing for that fruit, even though at the moment this is in contradiction with what you think about it yourself. In our first conversations we left all such matters undiscussed. We had plenty of other things to do rather than speculate about future developments. Perhaps that is the reason why these things are so concealed inside an obscure symbol.

When we make up the total balance, is there any reason for hope? Yes, there is. Several points enable us to think so:

- There is a plant that wants to grow.
- There is a knight who knows how to fight.
- There is a crocodile which is not given any chance to do harm and which flies around in the air.
- There is a girl, who eventually flies away in the shape of a dove.

On the other hand, a great many things still need to be done, and much will have to be changed in you if feelings of trust and hope for the future are to develop.

The Journey Begins on the Back of a Duck

A duck comes flying along. He is coming quite close to me and he is making a lot of noise. He claps his wings and chatters as if trying to tell me I have to go with him.

Now I see myself sitting on his back. I find this a bit frightening. I put my arms around his neck in order not to fall off. We are going high up in the sky. I hardly dare look down. Now we are up in the clouds, and I have a feeling as though we are changing into something different. We seem to have turned into a plane, and now we are turning into a balloon. Something goes wrong, the balloon catches fire. I am falling down and land on the doorstep of a church. I am not in any way hurt.

On either side of the entrance stands a devil. I get angry and I start hitting out at the devils. I make a terrible racket and smash them up completely. Now I enter the church. It is dark inside, but I can clearly see Christ on a cross. He has a funny head, a clown's head. I have had more than enough of all this. I take him from the cross, but when I have put him down he suddenly changes into a mole and the mole crawls away into the ground. Then I hack the cross into pieces as well, I sweep the whole lot together and put it all in the garbage can. Ugh, it is not very pleasant.

Another duck turns up. It seems to be the idea that I have to sit on his back and fly away with him. I can still feel the previous journey in my bones. I hear bells ringing. Again I see a church. The service has just finished, people are coming out. Then the picture changes. A great stream of water now comes pouring out of the church, and there is a canoe on the water. In the canoe sits a little girl with a baby on her lap. I take the baby from her. It seems I have something to do with this baby. The baby is happy.

Now the baby and I sit on the duck's back together. I am looking for a mother for this baby. Then suddenly I am standing by the canal. I see a ring glistening. It belongs to an Oriental princess wearing lots of jewels and with a little crown on her head. She beckons me. I approach and give the child to her.

For the third time a duck comes flying along. I don't have much desire for any more of these journeys. And yet it has to be. This time we go far away to the south. There we land on an island. I see a foot and when it changes it turns into a man. The man is busy hitting a little boy. This is too much. I give the man a wallop and he falls through a hatch and vanishes into the ground.

The little boy goes home on a bike. A momma with a white apron gives him a few good-natured little smacks. This is now my home as well. I am given chocolate milk and tea. The momma is nice. She asks me to tell her who I am and what is the matter with me. I don't quite know what to say and I almost choke. I tell her that I have lost my way and don't have a proper home. The momma sits down beside me and puts her arm around me. She strokes my back and my hair. It makes me feel much more peaceful. I am allowed to stay for as long as I like. I may also leave if I want to. I don't have to tell her anything more. I feel relieved.

I am still on the island. I am in a house where I see a mysterious object. It is a chest with a studded lid. When I look inside the chest I see a ring with a gold flower. I want to take it out, but the lid slams shut so I can't.

Then to my surprise I see the studs disappear from the lid and the chest opens again. The lid opens and shuts a few times. The ring is still inside but I dare not make another grab for it. When the lid opens again, a fat little man comes out of it, in a bowler hat and white gloves. The ring is on his finger on the outside of the glove. The man says, "I'll show you something funny." We walk quickly till we get to a big, expensive house. We enter a hall with a chandelier. The momma with the white apron is there too. She works here. Then I see the Oriental princess coming down the stairs. The little man shakes hands with her. I do the same. The princess then takes me upstairs with her. It's a posh place, that's for sure. I ask her what is the meaning of all this, because I don't really know what to do. First she asks me if I like it here and I say yes. Then she says, "You were to bring me the gold ring and I have something funny to show you."

Suddenly there is a little boy about two years old. "Look," she says, "I got him from you and I want to show you how well he is doing." The little boy comes up to me and plays with me. A moment later the princess feeds him from her breast. Then I give her the ring which the little man brought with him. And the ring begins to glitter.

IN SEARCH OF A MOTHER

There may be fairy tales in which a person flies on the back of a duck, but you don't expect that sort of thing to happen to yourself. So it must be strange to have this experience in one of your imaginations. But there is no escape: before you realize what is happening you find you are sitting on the back of a duck. At that moment you are no longer the only one who is in control of what goes on. There is another force besides, which seems to have its own plans for action. For the first time there is a clear indication here of a directing hand in the images, of which the ego figure has to take account. We are dealing here with an unambiguous case of abduction, for before you are aware of it you are already on your way, and, moreover, you have absolutely no idea of where the journey will be taking you. During this journey certain changes occur in the images; what is taking place inside your head is being made visible. A sequence of images expresses how frightening this adventure is for you. First is the image of sitting unprotected on the back of a duck. The duck becomes an airplane so as to offer you a little more protection. The fear of looking down causes clouds to form. The feeling of being unable to exercise control causes the airplane to change into an air balloon, and only the slightest whiff of fear is required to make the balloon catch fire.

Once you are down on the ground a signal is received indicating that such imaginal situations can all be overcome. You are standing safe and well on earth and nothing is broken.

All the same, the fear motif continues to play a part, because the entrance to the church, in which you have spent so many anxious moments, is flanked by two mighty devils. And then the time has come to make the knight inside you rise up, burst out in

anger and exorcise the devils. This is done with great thorough-
ness. It is as if the duck had picked on a place where something
needed to be put right. It was necessary to get rid of a number of
bad influences in your life. However, curbing these is not the end
of the mission, for in the church itself there are certain things that
need to be put right too. A Christ figure with a clown's head, that
is very ambiguous indeed. You do not hesitate for a moment and
you take him down from the cross. But for some reason you do
nothing more. The Christ figure vanishes like a mole under the
ground. He will no doubt return. Only that annoying cross is still
there. It arouses anger in you, this symbol of suffering, and you
want to get rid of it. Throw it in the garbage can!

When the duck appears once more, you are not pleased. Soon
afterward, there are bells ringing and another church appears; no
good can come of that. But look, strange things begin to happen;
a newly baptized child comes sailing along on the lap of a girl.
You have no doubt about what is being asked of you: you have to
pick up the baby and make sure that better arrangements will be
made for it. A mother must be found. Even though you are at
that moment not entirely aware of everything that is going on,
some very important things are happening right before your eyes.
Just think of it: a minute ago you were wreaking havoc in a
church, and almost immediately afterward a new sign of life has
appeared from this same church, in the form of a baby. Where are
you supposed to take this baby? The parents from the beginning
of the story, the witch and the monstrous gardener, are totally
unsuitable.

The duck helps out. It carries you and the baby away, and in
the middle of a busy city an Oriental princess is discovered and
found fit to be a mother to this new life. You might say that this is
the beginning of a renewal of your inner parent images. You are
permitted to have new feelings and very briefly to experience the
sense of having a home. This happens while you are sitting on the
back of a duck.

After the wicked father has been got rid of and another child
has found its way home, the time arrives when you yourself are

given an affectionate caress and are allowed to drink a cup of co-
coa. How simple and effective: "I feel peaceful and relieved." This
happens right after you had made it known that you had lost your
way and had no real home. From that moment everything begins
to acquire a hint of mystery. The ring with the golden flower
presages something good, but apparently your curiosity has to be
aroused first. There is a servant who shows you the way. What
could this very ordinary person be doing in such rich surroundings? The contrast is great. It is as if every effort were being made
to make it clear to you that you may expect something very special—and that the result will not be poor and shabby but that you
may hope for a costly reward. The herald of this is the little boy,
the one you recently entrusted as a baby to a princess. You see
that he is growing up healthily and is clearly in good hands.
What might all this mean with regard to you? For the moment it
is no more than a promise, and the reality looks very different. So
there is nothing for you to do but wait and see how the story will
develop.

The Journey Continues on Horseback

A train approaches. It stops at the station. It is an old-fashioned
train, one with a coal car. Something strange is going on. There
is someone lying on top of the coal car. He is lying on the coal,
tied up with ropes. I am standing close by. That man is dead!

Now I see a horse approaching. All alone. He does crazy
things: he goes to the man, licks him and starts to tug at his
coat. It is as if he is trying to say something. I believe I must
free the man, and so I start untying the ropes. It looks as if some
life is coming back to him. Then I lay the man on the back of
the horse, and I myself mount the horse as well. When we are
on our way I begin a conversation with the man. I ask him why
he was lying dead on that truck. He says he wanted to be dead
because all the time he was going around in circles and kept
having to throw coals on the fire. I know that feeling.

I notice that we have arrived at a castle. We enter the courtyard, without any formalities. A party is in full swing. The man sees an old friend and runs up to him. They fly into each other's arms, and I stand watching a bit timidly. They are having a good time and drink a pint of beer together. Now I am left all by myself.

In the courtyard there walks a knight. He is wearing a suit of armor and carries a sword in his hand. He comes toward me and beckons me to come with him. He mounts his horse, and I see that my horse is still there as well. We now move off together and we come to a wood. There are many more knights there. They are preparing themselves for battle.

In the middle of the circle there is a princess lying on the ground. It looks as if she is dead. When I come near, she moves. She gets up, falls upon my neck, and kisses me. She is happy. I find it all rather overwhelming. It seems to be the idea that I take her back to the castle. I do so, we sit on the brown horse together.

Then we arrive at the castle and sit down by an open fire. The princess sits very close beside me. She puts her arms around me and kisses me. I become confused by this and don't know what to do any more. I feel I ought to leave, so I go back to my horse.

One day I take a walk in the wild garden behind the castle. A man is picking berries there, very dark berries. His wife is making a drink out of them. It looks a bit suspicious. Poisonous. Who could she be mixing poison for? She is boiling the juice over a fire. I am quite sure it is intended for the princess.

I go back to the castle, because I must try to warn the princess. When I have found her and tell her what I have seen, she brushes it aside. She doesn't believe it. In the room I see rows of bottles all along the walls with exactly the same dark liquid in them. Then I pull her along with me outside and show her what is going on in the little house in the grounds behind the castle. But even then she does not believe me. She asks me to go back into the castle with her. When we arrive, a reception is taking place. The princess is now wearing very beautiful clothes. She is standing at the front and is being congratulated. To my surprise the bottles along the wall are all filled with a white drink. I don't understand what is going on. I myself am now standing at the far end of the line. And everyone is congratulating me too.

When I wake up and look out of the window, I see chickens in the courtyard. A girl of about seventeen, with curly hair, is busy feeding the chickens. I go outside and watch. High up in the tower a little door opens and a cockerel comes out. He begins to crow. I am irritated by this and call out to him to stop making such a noise.

Then I go for a walk and cross the castle moat, which looks dirty. It looks as if it is filled with pitch instead of water. There is a path running all around the castle. When I have walked some way along this path, the girl catches up with me. When I ask her what is the matter, she says I must come and help her feed the chickens. On the way back my attention is drawn to her hand. I see a ring glittering on it, but then I see it slipping from her finger and falling into the moat. There it remains, lying on the heavy pitch, so that I am able to pick it up. I give the ring back to the girl, and we continue our walk.

Having arrived back in the courtyard, I see the girl suddenly in a different place. She is holding a plank of wood in her hands that has the shape of a person. What a dry stick, I think. I don't like the look of it, and I take the plank away from her. She gets very angry with me and disappears into the castle.

The scene changes. I see market stalls. It looks a bit like a fair; there is a clown playing with rings. Then a knight comes riding along on horseback at great speed. He holds his lance pointed forward, goes straight for the clown, and stabs him to death. I am very upset at this: how could he do such a thing? Within seconds, the knight has vanished again. The clown flops down limply. I carry him indoors and lay him on a table. The girl comes in too. She has picked up the wooden plank and slides it under the clown. The clown is dead. The plank folds itself around him and becomes a coffin.

Sadly I look around and see a procession of women coming toward us, all of them dressed in black. The girl and I move to the head of the procession, and then the funeral begins. As the coffin is lowered into the grave, the lid begins to move. A baby comes out of it. Beaming and alive, it lies in the arms of its mother. I see alternately the clown and the baby and I think, "That is me."

In the courtyard a boy of about fourteen climbs over the castle wall. He is black all over. He must have fallen into the moat and now he runs across the yard and goes indoors. I feel fear inside me. Briefly the thought flashes through my mind that perhaps I ought to go and help to clean him up. I dare not look at him anymore, and I run away.

Now I am riding on my brown horse in a mountainous landscape. In front of me is a hooded cart with a man and a woman and a child. They are going to build a new life for themselves somewhere else. I want to do that too. Except I don't want to be their servant. I want to build up something for myself.

Something is going wrong now. The cart plunges down the mountainside, into the ravine. I tumble down as well, even farther down than the cart. At the bottom of the ravine I land in water. There are fishes in it, and a pointed rock sticks out above the surface. In the distance a canoe appears. When it comes closer I see the girl with the curly hair sitting in it. I think it is terrible that she should find me here like this. She takes me on board. I am angry that she has to rescue me, and I begin to cry. The girl is crying as well now and begins to comfort me. I lie down close beside her, but it is as though I am dead, I am so stiff. All the same, it is very nice sailing in the canoe with her.

We sail through a mountain gate and then I can see the sun and a beach. She gets dressed over her bathing suit and we walk on the beach together. We drink from a waterfall and see

another person there. It is a shepherd who looks like Christ. We
are invited to his hut. There I lie in a hammock and am being
cradled by the girl. We drink wine, and a moment later the girl
and I are walking on the beach again. Everything is wonderful.
It should always stay like this.

On the beach walks a black beetle. Ugh, what a horrid beast.
Away with it. I tread on it with my foot. The girl changes, her
face becomes a witch's face. This is all going badly wrong, I am
getting into a panic. I must try to make everything come right
again. The face is a mask and I pull and tug at it, to get rid of it.
It won't come off. I rush off in a great hurry to fetch the
shepherd. He reassures me and says it will be all right. He also
tries to take the mask off but he can't manage it either. Then he
gets angry and starts hitting out with a cudgel. I also pick up a
cudgel, and together we smash everything to smithereens. Then
I see a skeleton lying on the ground. We smash that to bits as
well. We then start to bury the whole lot. I am inconsolable. We
shovel earth all over everything, and then I see a flower coming
out of the earth. Attached to the stem of the flower there is a
little hand, and attached to the end of the hand there is a little
girl. First the flower is given to me, but I give it to the girl.
Shaken and upset, I walk back together with the man and
the girl.

Again there is a beach, but it is not by the sea. It is on the
bank of a river. I can hardly believe my eyes: horses are coming
out of the water and behind them a hearse. Everything is in
black, and men with black hats are sitting on top of the hearse.
Inside the hearse lies a princess, dressed entirely in white. She
has a crown of flowers in her hair. She is very young, no more
than about eighteen. The men drive to the village where I was
born. I am standing at the back of the hearse, with a bunch
of flowers in my hand. When I try to put the flowers on the
princess, she sits up, and then we are suddenly standing in the
road together. I say to her, "What were you doing in that
hearse?" She replies, "I was asleep." I am still surprised and say,
"But why were you lying in a hearse?" She says, "I wasn't dead"

and she laughs. We hold each other by the hand, we walk along
the road and laugh. I feel shy. When I mention that to her, she
says, "That doesn't matter." We talk for a while and she says she
likes me. I explain to her that I find it difficult to be with girls.
Then she starts romping about with me. I give her a few little
kisses and then I say, that's enough now. She gets on her bicycle
and waves. Wow, I feel excited and I am glad of a chance to
catch my breath.

The mountain landscape has come back again. An angel with
a halo is hovering around. I am not alone here. A dog is sniffing
around and barks. He is trying to get at something and pulls me
along on a lead. It makes me feel excited. Behind a bush I see a
girl with a handkerchief. I cannot see her very clearly and when
I come closer she has vanished. The dog is barking furiously.
He is by the water. It is a stream with very wild-running water.
The dog jumps into the stream and so do I. Swimming is
difficult but it is nice. Then the dog is on the shore again. He
has caught a hare. I shouldn't have allowed him to run loose. He
gobbles the animal up at once. He says he was hungry. Then he
says, "Let's walk on."

We cross a little bridge and arrive at a village. The first thing
we do is look for a café. There the dog laps up a bowl full of
water. The café owner is a fat man. At a table sit two old
women and a girl. I join them and I ask the girl whether she
was the girl I saw behind the bushes. She laughs. She is
wearing a little white hat, and that tallies. Then I ask her if she
would like to come out with me and she agrees. The two
women go on chattering. I ask her if she would like to go in a
canoe and she says she would. She sits in the front. The dog sits
on the bow.

I take the girl by the waist and I want to cuddle her. Then I
am necking with her while the canoe moves on regardless. I feel
wild. I can do anything I like. Then I pull the canoe onto the
bank. It is a grassy bank and there is a little shed. We lie in the
grass. The dog is running around. We are petting furiously. It is
very exciting. It makes me feel good. We romp and roll about.

There is beer and other drinks too. I am holding her in my arms. She has beautiful eyes. I am very surprised at myself. I didn't know I could do this. Now I am lying on my back looking at the sun, fantasizing a little.

Then we go back to the canoe. The dog is having fun. We row back, against the current, to the village. I take her to her house and then I sit on a terrace for a while to catch my breath.

A Sign of Life

That is what you might call the horse: a sign of life, and in that capacity the animal arrives just in time. The furnace stoker was at the end of his tether, going around in circles without the prospect of anything other than work. No hope of any encouragement. You get more and more stuck in a rut. Why should you try your best any longer? There is nothing that can give meaning to your life anyway. There is no friend, male or female, to whom you can devote yourself, and the days are dull. All contacts with other people have become overshadowed by fear and so there is nothing left for you to do but withdraw in your loneliness.

And as we have seen earlier, the horse comes to rescue his master. Not that the master knows anything about it. He doesn't even know that he is the master. This dawns on him only gradually. As a result of all the tugging and pulling at the stoker's coat, and the horse licking him, the message comes across that this man on the coal car must be set free. A few moments later you are on your way to a new future together. The instinctive first push toward this was given by the horse. The whole process of awakening consciousness that should now ensue will have to be accomplished by you, as a horseman. It is a process which leads you from one surprise to the next.

You arrive at a castle which you have never seen before and where festivities are in progress. The stoker is alive and kicking again, he joins a friend of his, and after drinking a pint of beer he is suddenly gone. You yourself are not taking any part in anything and you are left behind on your own. No friend for you.

You are predestined for something else. Your duties are at a higher level. This is made clear to you by a circle of knights who themselves have no time to look after the princess. That task has been reserved for you of all people, even though you are the least experienced in such matters. It is possible that there once lived a princess inside you, but she had never before manifested herself.[3] Now it seems that the time has come. When you approach her, over there in the circle, she suddenly gets up and throws herself about your neck. This is something that can happen to anybody, and it is now happening to you: namely, that the female part of yourself has emerged. Your task now consists in uniting this part with what you already knew before. If you succeed, new possibilities will become available to you, particularly in your contact with other people. Perhaps also in your contacts with women, but we cannot be altogether sure about that yet. At this moment you still have a very different opinion about it, so we shall have to wait and see how these things develop.

All these changes begin at once. The unconscious part of the horse rider, represented by the princess, takes the initiative. She falls about his neck and kisses him and when they arrive at the castle she even becomes rather over-insistent and this is more than he is able to cope with at this moment. He has to go back to his horse for a while. But in fact, it was the horse that arranged the whole thing in the first place. It is therefore reasonable to expect that the story which began here will be continued according to plan.

As it happens, the horse rider has already been touched by a spark, for a moment later, when he thinks he has discovered a plot against the princess, he does not hesitate to take up his knightly duties. Once again we see a gardener and his wife engaged in sinister activities; they are mixing poison, by which they hope, just like the witch from the beginning of the story, to prevent the future from happening. They will not succeed. In the first place, the horse rider tries to frustrate their plan by warning the princess, but he is unable to persuade her. She does not believe him. However, she proves stronger than he expected. She can make things change into their opposites, and it is just as well that she has this ability because her task is going to be exactly that. As for him, he starts off at the far end of the line, but he is being congratulated nevertheless. How strange, to stand there being congratulated and not knowing why. Unless you believe that fate can be reversed. Perhaps that belief is born here.

The following scene forms the starting point for treatment of the sexual problem. While the girl is feeding the chickens, the cockerel begins to make his presence known, high up in the tower. You might say he is blowing his own horn, and he can be heard clearly, even though, to be frank, his crowing meets with little favor. He ought to keep quiet, because he is disturbing the peace.

The girl with the curly hair, however, is imperturbable. She comes to fetch him back from his walk and then does something which he does not like at all. She is acting very demonstratively with that wooden plank of hers. It ends in a squabble, though not for long, for immediately afterward there follows a scene with a clown, a scene that is difficult to understand. The clown is stabbed to death and buried along with the wooden plank. It is as though it is suggested that these two parts of the persona had better be put out of action. With regard to the clown, it actually fits in with what you yourself did earlier to the Christ figure, who also had a clown's head. You must have something against the clown. The way has now been cleared for the baby, as a symbol of new life.

Everything has been shaken up: the princess has prepared the way for the encounter with the girl with the curly hair. The various complications have contributed to the forging of a bond. What about all the other feelings you are aware of having? The knowledge that you feel attracted to younger boys must surely still be there? And the fact that for this reason you felt a tremendous inner struggle? This aspect of yourself is also presented in an image, albeit very fleetingly: a boy climbs over the castle wall, covered in pitch, which lay as a turbid mass in the moat. What should I do, what do I want, what do I fear? The boy runs to the other side and you run away in order not to have to meet him. Presumably this wasn't just a trivial decision taken on the spur of the moment. At least it seemed as though the horse rider was planning to leave for good. He joins a small family with the aim of building a new existence somewhere else. The castle has become too unsafe a position. One thing is clear: you don't want to be a fool. What you want is to build up a new life, something for yourself. But what can be done about the story that has just been set into motion? It follows its course regardless. After all, you are still riding your brown horse, aren't you? The horse will see to it that the course taken thus far will be continued.

The flight is interrupted dramatically. Everything suddenly topples into a ravine. The language of the images can hardly be called mild. Although the fall into the ravine does not lead to injury, the experience is nevertheless a painful one. The initial plan cannot be carried out. For the time being, no cosy little cottage for you.

Your path is deflected, and you are led once again to the girl with the curly hair. If it was unavoidable to meet her, you would have preferred not to do so in a state of near-drowning. On the other hand, it is doubtful whether in that case you would ever have gone out of your way to look for her. Luckily, you are welcomed with real sympathy, and so the sun breaks through the clouds again. Together you are washed up on the beach near the shepherd, and for a very brief time you are in paradise. Why then should this idyll be disturbed yet again? We can only guess at the reason. To do so it is necessary to investigate the image of the black beetle, to discover what this insect signifies in other situations.[4] It might represent your worry about the growth of feelings that are not yet allowed to exist, for instance sexual feelings. The image would then imply that you are unconsciously reproaching yourself for these feelings. The beetle is therefore immediately trampled into the ground. At the same time, however, the idyllic scene has vanished as well. Once again, the witch appears. This is a heavy punishment, with which you must learn to come to terms. Maybe it would be sensible to allow more scope to the things that go on in your mind and to give expression to these in your encounters.

In a symbolic way this is exactly what you now set out to do:
you settle once and for all with what went wrong just now so you
can start with a clean slate. It is not a clean slate, though. It is
more than that, it is a slate with a flower on it and a moment later
with a little girl on it as well. You have to learn something that
was interrupted very early in your life. To do so, you receive a
flower, which you give to the little girl. The lesson is soon learned.
The flower is the symbol for certain feelings, and these you give to
the girl. When you were on the beach this could not yet happen,
but now the way has been cleared for it. Let us have a look at the
result. The horses walk in front. Behind them a hearse emerges
from the water. Is is hardly possible to think of a greater contrast.
Water is the symbol of life-energy, of the source of life, and out of
the water rises a hearse. In the hearse lies a princess, and she
appears to be dead. A moment later it turns out that she was
merely asleep. So what was she, dead or asleep? We can draw
a comparison here. When we become conscious of something,
something that was dead comes to life again. So the princess is
awakened for a second time. You wake her by giving her not one
flower but a whole bunch. You obviously intend to show her
more of your feelings. No sooner thought than done, and you tell
her about your shyness with girls. And when it appears that she
respects these feelings, without allowing herself to be inhibited in
her actions, you are able to take the initiative and you kiss her a
few times. And then you have learned enough for one day.

A new guide appears and this time it is the dog. This becomes
a rather more personal relationship than the one you had with the
horse, and as a result the story as a whole begins to take a more
personal turn. What is clear from the start is that the dog reflects
something of what goes on in the mind of the master, and vice
versa. Yet the dog is always a step ahead. He is out for adventure
and runs where his nose leads him. You yourself are far more uncertain, so you will have to sniff things out very carefully. Just as
suddenly as the dog catches a hare, so you plunge straight into a
café and invite a girl out. How are you suddenly brave enough to
do that? It doesn't matter. Maybe you learned it from the dog. At

any rate, crazy things are happening and I can't follow all of it. But never mind, perhaps the fact that the dog chased after a hare will provide an explanation.

For this reason we will keep an eye on the dog for a bit longer. He has meanwhile caught the hare. If we take as our starting point that nothing in these stories is a coincidence, it would make sense to examine what the hare as an animal-symbol could possibly represent.

The hare is of highborn origin. In mythology, the hare used to be linked with the moon and therefore with the moon-goddess, who guaranteed fertility and the constant renewal of life.[5]

In a narrower sense the hare was seen as a sexual symbol, and in this respect the fact that the dog eats the hare forms a sort of introduction to the events that follow.

But the hare also stands for fear, because of its ability to sleep with its eyes open, and this, together with the speed with which it can run, enables us to say a few things about fear. In this particular case the fear-hare is eaten up, and when this happens the fear has gone and you can return to action.

The dog shows his master the way and shows him how to deal with fear. Instead of allowing yourself to be brought to a halt on the way toward inner renewal, it is possible to sidestep the fear.

In the café the dog laps up a bowlful of water. He is thirsty and it seems that you are thirsty too, when you see the girl, the same girl as you thought you had seen behind the bushes. Your thirst is of a very different kind and you head straight for the girl and suggest that the two of you go in search of adventure together.

And indeed it turns out to be a great adventure. What has happened to your shyness? There is nothing left of it. The fear-hare has been gobbled up. In the canoe, with the dog sitting on the bow, you can even stop steering. The canoe continues on its way all by itself and everything points to it that this first love adventure will be a great success.

Romping and fondling in the grass. Drinks arriving from somewhere. "I didn't know I could to this." And it is true, in reality you can't, not yet, but it won't be long. The inner revolution, which has been in progress for quite a long time already, ever since the first imagination to be precise, is now gathering momentum.

And it appears that even such explicit symbolism has to be seen in a broader context. There is much more at stake. There is an inner revolution going on, through which the fear that still threatens to block your path must be overcome.

The future, which seemed blocked, has now been made free. You can start to fantasize about what you are going to do with it.

The Old Man and His Sketch Book

A bird is sitting in front of me. It is the duck. It seems that we are about to go off flying again. The trip does not take long this time. We are already on the descent again, and as we go down we dive underneath a hat. Hey, wasn't there somebody under that hat? Yes, I can see now, there is a very old man under it, with gray hair and wearing a very long white robe. His shoulders are stooping and he leans on a stick. I help him along and ask who he is. "I am a wise old man," he says. "Great, maybe I can ask him some things," I think.

It occurs to me that I always feel very anxious when I am near older women and also near women of my own age. I ask the old man if he knows why this is so. He says there is no need to be anxious. Then he points, and I see a girl standing near by. "She is a nice girl," he says. Meanwhile he strokes my hair.

I want to ask him whether it would really be possible for me to fall in love with a girl. I feel so uncertain about it. The old man clearly understands what I wanted to ask. He holds me closely against him and I see that at the same time he is comforting a very small baby. It is a naked little boy, about two or three years old. I have a feeling as though I am that little boy. "This little boy has been very cold," he says.

Then he points to the stained glass window of a church. There is a picture of a cockerel in it. You must go to the Virgin Mary, he says. I ask him to come with me, because I always used to be very frightened in church. He says he'll come. We enter the church together.

Inside the church it is very dark. I see another old man, with a big beard and a mean face. Water is being poured on his head. A kind of baptism presumably. Now I also see the face of a black woman with white hair. The wise man is with me. I tell him that I am afraid of these people and that I feel as if I want to start a fight. He says, "You'd better not do that, you'd better take a careful look at them. Maybe they have something for you or know something that will be useful to you."

Now I see an altar covered with a white sheet and with a beautiful crown on it. The man with the horrid face puts the crown on the head of the black woman. I say that I like the crown very much but that I am scared of the black face. The woman says she can see I am scared. I ask her whether she has something for me. She does not reply. Then I take her by the hand. It is a beautiful hand and I stroke it. Suddenly the black mask falls away, but there is a hideous face under it. I stroke the ugly face. Then it suddenly becomes very beautiful. She says, "You have made me better." I say that I can now see her better too. At that moment the big open mouth of an animal, of a crocodile, goes past.

I quickly huddle up against the old man. His face also keeps changing but I trust him all the same. "What should I do now?" I say. He picks up a book with pictures and shows me a drawing. I see two figures in turn: a little boy and a man of about thirty who is in great pain. The little boy is laughing.

The old man asks if I would like to go on a bike ride with him. He himself is at this moment riding a very old bike. A ridiculous sight, actually. I tell him I always feel awful when I am on a bike. "Why should that be?" he asks. I say I always feel that I don't belong. He asks whether I think this is still the case, because those awful feelings are no longer there all the time. "That is true. I can really enjoy myself now, but there are still a lot of things I dare not do. I would like to try those. I am still rather frightened of going outside." He says, "That may well

remain so for a long time, but it doesn't get you any further." I
ask if he will come to the bakery with me. He says that's okay,
and so we go on the bike together. "You can tell me all about
what is going on inside you," he says, "the others won't hear."
When we enter the bakery he says, "What is happening?" "I feel
warm and excited but not afraid," I tell him. The baker's wife
comes forward and serves me. I want some apple turnovers and
some rolls and my mind is occupied with the various things in
the glass show case, and I am no longer scared. "This is how it
should be, you're going to be all right," says the man. The
woman talks to me. I grow warm all over, at the thought that I
can do this! I feel very happy. That this should be possible!

The man smiles. I can cry as much as I like. The woman does
not notice anything.

Now a hand and a pencil can be seen. The pencil is drawing
a small flower. A pigeon comes along and flies away with the
flower. I follow him. The pigeon gives the flower to a girl with
a large hat. When I go up to the girl she gives me the flower. I
ask her if she knows the pigeon, because she waved to him.

"Yes," she says, "he always brings me something nice."

"Are you pleased with the flower?" she asks. "Yes," I say,
"but I feel unsure. There is something behind it which makes
me not altogether trust it. I still feel hesitant, I still can't bring
myself to think that something is really beautiful and to be
confident that things are really okay with me."

Then she gives me a large bunch of roses. It brings a lump to
my throat. She says, "You have earned them." I realize that it is
upsetting me and I just stand there looking at the flowers. She
asks me if I am finding it difficult to feel good. I look at her and
see a kitten lying on the brim of her hat. The kitten is purring
contentedly. That is exactly the kind of feeling I am unable to
have. She says the kitten feels at home with her.

Then the old man appears again. He has a doll in his hand. I
tell him about the woman and the roses. Then he gives the doll
to me. I am not too sure what to do with it. It is quite a nice
doll. The old man strokes its hair. Then he says that the doll is

the small child in me which feels good. "And when it feels bad you notice it in your tummy," he says. "You have to trust that little child inside you."

"But I thought I was supposed to be big and strong," I object.

"That is not enough," he says. "You must be able to feel good, and then you can do anything."

"I'd like to try that," I say.

Then he leafs through his sketch book. He points at a picture of an old-fashioned lamp on the ceiling. It is the lamp we used to have at home, when I was little. I see the little boy from earlier on.

"What do you know about him?" asks the man.

"He's a nice little boy," I say, "but he is scared and restless."

"If you think he is nice, then surely you can trust him?"

"Yes, I can, but he should have had more warmth."

"You can give him warmth, can't you?"

I do so, and the child is happy. I see he is thinking up plans for the future. I am glad to have such a happy little boy with me. That way I myself can make something of my life too.

We ought to visit each other more often.

THE CORE OF THE SELF

With the appearance of the Wise Old Man we have entered a decisive stage in the development. He is regarded as one of the figures that can be found in the immediate vicinity of the core of the Self. From the description you give of him, it is clear that he does not shrink from behaving comically. He is dressed in a long white robe, a sign of his dignity, but at the same time he is riding an old-fashioned bicycle. He is the sort of person one ought to have a certain respect for, because his wisdom is great, while at the same time he is someone with whom it is possible to have an ordinary conversation.

The relation of trust between you has come about very quickly and this enables you very soon to start talking about one of the things you find most puzzling. After your exciting adventures with the girl in the meadow, certain questions have risen in your mind. Would it be possible, after all, for you to fall in love with a girl? Are all the things you had assumed about yourself in this respect not true? Your fear when meeting women and girls is surely still there? I think you are very brave to speak about these things so directly. The "old fellow," as you call him, is not easily shocked. He takes the bull by the horns without any ado. He shows you a girl so that you can get used to the idea, and he makes it clear that there is no need for the little boy inside you to be afraid.

And then he sends you straight to the Virgin Mary. We must consider this carefully, because a church is not the place where you have your best memories, and to you Mary does not have a trustworthy face. Everything in the church has been overshadowed by the anxious moments you used to spend there in the company of your parents. You were always afraid that something might happen to them there, to your parents, and that you would then not know what to do.

In some way or other your trust will have to be restored, before you can get any further with the other problem. "Go and see if she has something for you," says the wise man. She has something indeed, but before you can receive it you will have to change your attitude toward her. Your tender solicitude makes her face change and now you can see her differently.

For the second time you see the dragon or the crocodile near Mary and it is as though this animal, as a representation of the threatening aspect of the feminine, is about to lose its sharp teeth.[6]

The way the wise old man tackles the problem is amazing. He does not disguise anything but confronts you directly with your difficulties. On the other hand he does not abandon you to cope on your own. Whenever you succeed in overcoming a small part of your fear, you feel better as a result. And when the threats become too great, his reassuring presence is always a help to you. The old man, as a representation of the core of the Self, steers toward a rearrangement of the past, thereby clearing the way for all the things that cause you so much worry in the daily reality of your life.

It is as if you yourself are now ready for it as well, for you are telling him of your difficulty in entering stores and doing shopping. Enough trust has been built up for you to go to him with very concrete problems. Once again it is demonstrated how resolute a person he is. First he asks you a number of informative questions about what exactly these unhappy feelings are like, of not belonging and so on. Then he suggests you tackle them. In order to do so it is first of all necessary to find a good part of yourself. In some way or other he knows that you don't have these miserable feelings all the time. There are times when you are able to enjoy yourself. Armed with this strong side of yourself, you set out together.

Once again the motto is: "Don't fuss, just get on with the job." Your feelings of anxiety occur mostly when you are imagining what happens at moments when you are getting stuck, when you have a feeling as though you can't escape. You get into a terrible panic then, and you'd like nothing better than to sink into the ground, without anyone knowing. The wise man says, "That may well remain so for a long time, but it doesn't get you any further." This gives you the bright idea of asking him to go to the bakery with him. He agrees and reminds you that he exists only inside you, and that therefore nobody else can see him. So you can talk to him without any worry, because nobody will notice anything. You can talk to him about all the awful feelings that keep rising up inside you. The strange thing though, is that those feelings don't come any more. His invisible presence is sufficient to reassure you and you are therefore able to concentrate on all the nice food you want to buy. You are even able to notice the friendly face of the baker's wife. Everything is going smoothly.

"That's how it should be," says the man. Of course, now you can enter the bakery with a quiet mind. Whenever an unhappy feeling arises, you can talk about it with him. Naturally, not all your problems will be solved all at once. You have had far too many unfortunate experiences. Step by step you will be able to get rid of the problems and with each good experience your self-confidence will grow.

At this point the earlier story is picked up again. The man makes it clear to you that boys don't only have to be brave and strong. There is room for the little boy inside them as well. Indeed, the little boy is very important, because he still knows what it is to have fun, as long as you look after him properly. Without the little boy you would turn into a mere roughneck. Warmth is what you need.

The Unknown Alphabet

In front of me crawls a snake with a three-forked tongue. It reminds me of the pain I have been feeling ever since I met the girl. In reality, I mean. She was nice to me and yet it gave me a stabbing pain. The snake looks menacing, but I look steadily at him and that keeps him quiet. The old man is near by. With his stick he is keeping the snake at bay. I tell him what is on my mind and I say I want to do something about it. Then the stick that the man is holding changes into a dung-fork with three prongs, and he is making stabbing movements with it in my direction. I don't understand. It is not like him at all to do that. "That is exactly it," he says, and he gives me the fork. "This thing is yours," he says. "You can feel those stabs coming at you, but they are your own and you can do something good with them. You don't need to worry about the pain, because you can do something with it." I tell him that I sense vaguely what he means, but that I would like to do something about it.

Meanwhile the fork has become a spade in my hands. Wait a moment, that means I can hack the snake to pieces and shovel it under the sand. The old man nods approvingly.

Then he takes up his picture book again and turns to a page with trees and shrubs and with a very fat goose on it. The goose tries to fly but it is so heavy that it keeps falling to the ground. I am supposed to go on a journey with this goose. We manage to get up in the air and soon afterward land in the water. We can make better progress there. The bird chatters profusely, but I tell him I want to work on this pain of mine. "Come along then," says the goose and points to a door which is locked. The keys hang beside it. I open the door and all at once all manner of things come rolling out. Lots of little glass pebbles. Very sharp. Lots of little diamonds, right in front of my feet. I feel them at my bare feet and they produce the same sharp pain.

Meanwhile the goose has swum away. I want to enter by the door but I can't get across the mountain of pebbles. Nor can I pick them up with my bare hands. What am I to do? Suddenly I see a beautiful girl approaching, with a glittering ring on her finger. She has an emery cloth with her and starts rubbing one of the pebbles to make it smooth. She gives it a lovely shape. I tell her I think she is making it very lovely but that at this rate it will take us five years to finish. Then I remember I had a shovel with me earlier on. I pick it up again and shovel the pebbles to one side. Now that I have seen what the girl did with them, they don't hurt so much any more.

Behind the door it is pitch-dark. The girl has just finished another pebble and she gives it to me to take with me, because it sheds a small amount of light, for indoors. I haven't nearly finished with that black den in there yet. It gives me a horrible, dark feeling again. I have to step across a pile of junk. Lots of branches covered in white mildew. Yet I want to go on. Nobody has been here for years. Here and there burns a candle. On a stone slab lies a person with a cloth over him. It is a boy of about fifteen. The woman removes the cloth from him. The boy is alive and I see his hard-on. I put the cloth over him again and the woman gives him a hug. I ask the boy where he has been. The woman replies that he has missed a lot but that she has now woken him up. He says that everything has stood still. He asks me where I have come from. I tell him about the rubbish I had to step across and what it was like outside. Then he says he

wants to go in the opposite direction. The three of us continue
on our way. He walks between us.

It becomes lighter ahead. I can see a princess over there. She
is wearing the glass pebbles in her hair and on her dress. The
boy rushes into her arms. She puts a long cloak around him.
Then we walk on. I myself am now that boy. The princess
points behind her. Everything I have left behind is there.
Then she points ahead. In front of us is a vast landscape. She
says, "How quiet you have become!" That is true. It is too
overwhelming. I cannot quite take it in yet. I want to ask the
old man about it. This time he is carrying a very small book
with him, with letters in it. They look like a kind of Roman
letters which I can't read. I say to him, "I can't read any of that!"
He says, "You can learn to read such letters." I tell him that the
princess and I are standing in front of a vast landscape together
and that it would be a great help to me if only I could manage to
take a few steps. I ask him if he could please give me a little
push. Instead, he gives me an old lamp to take with me. Very
briefly I glimpse a tall, pointed mountain. I feel an urge to start
climbing again, as I have so often felt before. But I don't do it
this time. I don't have to prove myself any more. I prefer to stay
on ground level. A feeling of tranquility fills me.

THE SHARP EDGES OF HAPPINESS

There are so many things to be noticed in a story like yours. If
you had to search for the exact interpretation, there would be
room for a great deal of hairsplitting. Let us resist that temptation
and simply concentrate on the things that strike us most. This is
what you yourself have to do all the time in that fabulous inner
world of yours. At every moment you are faced with the question:
what am I to do with this, and what does what I see do to me? It
is the same with me when I listen to you and hear about all your
adventures.

Well then, my attention is drawn by the three-forked tongue of the snake and the three prongs of the dung fork. Admittedly, this is partly because I have read something about it. We will speak of that later. Meanwhile, the old man nods with approval when you chop the snake to pieces. In order to do so you have used the tool that was handed to you, and this is, of course, what matters. The fact that a snake has been lost is of no great consequence. The old man knows better than we do that the snake cannot really be got rid of. The snake is eternal and is bound to turn up again somewhere or other. Snakes often represent life that renews itself. Its special attribute in this case is the three-forked tongue. The importance of this is underlined by the old man when he points a three-pronged fork at you. In India this trident is the attribute of the god Shiva and has a very special significance. It stands for past, present, and future; or for the basic attributes of the perceivable world: Becoming, Being, and Decaying.[7] Seen in this light, the three-forked tongue, with which your story here begins, is a succinct summary of what you are about to experience immediately afterward. You are busy taking leave of the past. In the past you were accustomed to sorrow and pain from which it was impossible to free yourself. In the inner world, however, grief and pain are no incontrovertible facts. "You can do something with it," says the old man. This is a difficult message, because we are not used to such possibilities. Quite rightly, you ask him whether you are really allowed to do something with it, so that you may experience the truth of what he says.

The fat goose, which finds it so hard to get off the ground, is a good guide. You yourself also find it hard to get off the ground. One thing is certain, the goose is not stupid. He knows how to break through to the future, where there are new possibilities, and he has hung the keys beside the door in advance.

The key to the future, which is here being given to you, leads you into a cave. That is the place where we can find the abandoned parts of our Self. When you have told the goose that you want to do something about your pain, which has accompanied your feelings of happiness, he shows you the way to this cave. So that is where the answer must lie. You find a piece of yourself there: the boy of fifteen, just about to enter upon sexual maturity, had been left behind in the unconscious Self and that was why your own growth remained deprived of that essential element. It is understandable that you have not yet overcome your confusion about these things. In mythology, the cave was the place where the goddess of nature lived, and to judge by your story she lives there still. Now that you have succeeded in finding the entrance to this cave, she proves able to awaken the boy in you to new life, so that you can assimilate him into your existence. That is what you can do about your pain: make sure that the boy will once again become a part of your conscious Self, and then the pain will gradually disappear.

Together with the woman from the cave you take the boy outside and, sure enough, a fusion then takes place. "I myself am now that boy," you say, and as you say it an essential change has occurred in your life. You will have to get used to the idea that from now on this happiness can be yours. Whether all the pain will now have gone for ever is another question, for happiness is a very vulnerable possession and you have to have courage to live with it.

The vast landscape in front of you immediately overwhelms you. It is too immense to comprehend all at once. So much space and air to breathe in, it is too much. Quickly back to the old man to ask him if he can give you a little push. But the masterful therapist has other things on his mind. You were a little disappointed by that. You are fobbed off with an old lamp and as an honest-to-goodness Boy Scout you know that such lamps do not cast their light very far. What use is it to you? But you soon discover that the old man's wisdom is operating here too. The lamp does not give much light and that is a good thing. It means that you can see no further ahead than one meter at a time. Step by step is his motto. Don't try to conquer the whole landscape all at once and storm up the first mountain you see.

This is a fairly random point at which to leave you. The instructive process in our imaginal world is never at an end. For the scope of this book it seems a good point to say goodbye. The road to the future is open and I wish you all the best on your journey.

Dealing with Inner Images

I knew that I sometimes had dreams from which I later remembered images, usually of concrete experiences and situations. I was also familiar with daydreams and fantasies. But I was not aware that I would be able to see images or representations and make them up myself. It was therefore a strange sensation to close my eyes and start seeing all kinds of fantastic images just like that. Especially at the beginning I needed to concentrate very hard, because the images often changed or faded very rapidly. It was a great help to relate aloud what I saw, to give descriptions and say what sort of feelings attended each image.

It is not altogether clear to me whether while I am telling my story I am actually directing the imaginations. Even when I am not relating anything I still follow the developments and see new images appearing all the time, but then they do not so easily form a story. It can happen that I receive a lot of very different images, following one after another, which do not seem to have anything to do with one another. On the one hand, I can sometimes exercise influence and intervene in situations. For instance, I was able to stop a witch from carrying out her evil designs on a child. On the other hand, at a given moment I wanted to see the face of a girl I was able to see only in outline, but however hard I concentrated, I could not see her face. At another time I was in a cemetery and wanted to get away. I did, but then I came back to it by a roundabout way without wanting to.

The images evoke all kinds of feelings: fear, grief, happiness, security. It was a reassuring thought to have someone near me

who could give me instructions, especially when I was getting
frightened. The most important remarks spoken to me were:
"Can you make contact with ——?" or: "Can you talk to him or
her?" By making contact with a person of whom I was
frightened, I became aware of my own strength. In this way I
learned to slay monsters and render witches harmless.
Afterward I would have a sense of relief.

These helpful remarks caused me to be more actively
involved with the images. With the result that I began to feel
more confident in looking at them and was able to view them
more calmly and with detachment. Being involved with images
is a very intensive activity. Sometimes I am extremely tired after
only fifteen minutes. Then I lose my concentration and the
images start running into one another or they become vague,
and then I stop. The effect the images have on me is the same as
a dream. After unpleasant images I feel bad and if they have
been pleasant I feel moved. I have noticed that examining the
images had a systematic influence on my dreams. It is as if I
were making a fresh journey through my life, starting in early
childhood and gradually moving toward puberty and beyond.
The thoughts I had during the day also had their parallels in the
images. So there was an air of repetition about it all, except that
I can now exercise influence on what happens, which used not
to be the case.

The events that occurred in fairy-tale-like surroundings, in
castles and among knights and princesses, would suddenly
alternate with very concrete situations, such as I had
experienced in the past. Even when I had completely forgotten
them, I was right back in the middle of them. They were as real
and clear as if they were happening here and now, with the
same smells, sounds, and feelings as before. Unbelievable. With
the only difference that this time I was able to be more active.
Sometimes I would even be terribly aggressive, but also
persuasive. I was able to say what was on my mind and make
the situations more bearable for myself. Many of these
flashbacks had to do with my old home. At first this confused

me, but because both the therapist and I wrote everything down, I slowly began to see a very clear line in the events. Especially at the beginning my images were very unhappy, so that I started to think that they were doing me more harm than good. The therapist then told me that the images would gradually become better. This was explained to me with the aid of developments in the imaginations. Sometimes the explanations were very surprising, so that I became more and more enthusiastic and also more curious. Writing then down was helpful, but from time to time it was an awful chore as well, because it made me experience everything all over again. It wasn't until much later that I could bring myself to read the stories again.

2 – SETTLING AN INNER CONFLICT

The Boy with the Fair Hair

On a parking lot stands a minibus with young people in it. A boy with fair hair beckons me to go with them. After driving for a while we arrive at a campsite in the dunes near the sea. A tent is put up, but nobody talks to me. I feel myself getting angry. It is as if I do not belong. When it becomes clear that there is nothing I can do about it, I decide to leave.

The boy with the fair hair follows me. It is important to me that he should understand me. The boy is sad. I realize that my anger is more like sadness too. I have to explain something very important to him, which makes me very anxious. From a distance I now see myself talking to him. I am in two places at once and so I am able to tell him something without being frightened. It seems to give me much relief. It all looks very self-evident and easy, yet I cannot get any closer. Quite the contrary, I am walking away from him now.

My path leads straight into the sea. The waves wash over me and I arrive in a large hall under water. There I see a circle of black figures coming to warn me. I must go away from there, because otherwise the whole house will collapse. Through an opening I get out of the hall, but here too there are black figures that want to touch me. I am frightened out of my wits and I hit out and lash about me, because I don't want them to touch me. They won't stop, until I escape from the circle and slowly drift upward. On the beach I climb back into myself and spend the night in a tent.

The next day I walk into the dunes again. There is a large

flock of black birds pointing the way to a dip in the dunes. There lies the fair-haired boy, he is wounded. When I come closer he takes on a terrifying appearance. When I shrink back, his face becomes ordinary again. He stretches out his arms toward me, but I stand as if nailed to the ground. There is a thick wall around me, which prevents me from getting closer to him, and so I cannot explain anything either.

Dejectedly I walk away and a moment later I am in a cellar. Through a little window I can see lots of legs walking down the street. The people are walking behind a cart with black birds sitting on it. It is a hearse. The fair-haired boy is being buried. At the cemetery he stands beside me and explains that it concerns a part of him which has caused a wall to exist between us. From now on he will always be accessible to me, but I may also go away if I wish. I cannot lose him again.

The Dividing Wall

At the beginning of this therapy I was hoping for concrete solutions to concrete problems. I had been working on this for several years but the only thing I achieved was that it became easier to talk about my problems. I had hardly found any solutions. My feelings had become strengthened and had come to the surface more. But I still wasn't able to live with them. I continued to find everything pointless and useless, especially myself.

I then allowed myself three months to try out this new therapy. I found it difficult to believe that the images that occurred to me might have an influence on my daily life. I knew from books what you had to do to be able to live together with other people, but I could not feel it personally and I also couldn't believe that people really loved me. What I experienced in the images and in the stories in which I took part was detached from the rest of my life. I knew that the symbols were very ancient and that the theory had been thoroughly worked

out, but all the same, I kept being assailed by doubts. In the end
I still had to do it all by myself and I felt rejected.

The theory about the unconscious seemed very plausible to
me, but mostly as it applied to other people, not to myself. That
is why it took a long time before I was able to draw connections
between the "fantasies" and my daily life. Very gradually I
began to see and feel what certain symbols stood for. The theory
then became less important, I began to discover that the events
of the week influenced the images, and the other way around.

But my doubts were stubborn, and my problems remained as
they were. At some moments I was even finding life more
difficult than before. My panic and anxiety increased. There
were times when I no longer dared be alone. In all my twenty-
eight years I had never, as a woman on my own, found life so
difficult. One thing was sure, I could no longer deny that the
images were of influence.

THESE OUTPOURINGS OF yours from the early days make it clear
to me that things weren't going very well between us. There was
a wall between you and other people and therefore also between
you and me. Not a wall of hostility, built on purpose. More a necessary evil. Without that wall you would at that moment not have
been able to cope. It was an essential protection, but a very unsatisfactory one, and a great obstacle to us in our efforts to work
together successfully. It couldn't be helped, because it was obviously not feasible to get rid of the wall just for one hour of
therapy in the week. Our working relationship is therefore per-
force somewhat imperfect at the moment, and we can only hope
that it will gradually improve.[1]

This problem of the dividing wall between you and other people
is what we are here concerned with. The imagination about the
boy with the fair hair makes it painfully clear: you would love to
make contact, but for reasons that are for the moment incomprehensible you are prevented from doing so by a huge barrier of
fear. The fact that you so badly wanted to make contact was

probably the reason why you felt you had to explain something to him, so that there would be no misunderstanding between you. What exactly it was that had to be explained will perhaps remain a secret for ever. At any rate you yourself never found out what was said there, and neither did I. Maybe the boy will be able to tell you one day.

Here then is the strange possibility that an unconscious part of you transmits a message while the conscious part watches from a distance. You know that your message has come across and that it has brought relief, no more. And you had no feelings of anxiety when this happened, because the operation was probably necessary.[2]

For a time there is a certain duplication. A moment later you leave and then something threatens to go wrong. The dark beings you see moving across the wallpaper at home at night also come to spoil your life here. They threaten to touch you and this makes you feel sick with fear. Just in the nick of time you see a chance to talk to them briefly; you have to rise to the surface, because otherwise the whole house will collapse. That is to say, the dark figures make you fear that your whole personality will cave in and this is too great a threat for you to continue your journey under water. The unknown terrain down below will for the present remain unknown to you and therefore also unloved.

The next morning the black birds are there. They introduce a funeral. In this inner world, dying and being buried do not have the same meaning as they have outside; they represent a return into the unconscious, and although this implies a form of leave-taking, there is also the possibility of a return.

So this is what the boy tells you: the part that creates a division between you is relegated to the unconscious, because otherwise it would prevent all movement. For the time being you two can make contact only in a certain way. Of course this is unsatisfactory, but for the moment it has to be. Perhaps there will be a better opportunity later, once the barrier of fear has been broken down.

A *Grandfather in Shirt Sleeves*

The weather is sunny and I see vast wheat fields all around.
There are many bees and dragon flies in the air. Beyond a bend
in the road a lake is just visible, with lots of reeds growing along
the bank. When I come closer I see a jetty and a little boat
moored by it.

I decide to get into the boat and take a little trip. In the
middle of the lake is an island with lots of trees. Standing
among the trees is a small shed. My boat drifts onto the beach.
On the shore I hear the sound of a saw. I am rather frightened of
going there.

When I arrive at the shed I see an old man with curly hair, in
shirt sleeves. He is smoking a pipe and looks like a grandfather.
There is a bench nearby on which I can sit. The man has almost
finished chopping logs for the fire. He looks as if he is waiting.

I ask who he is. A wind has come up and the man now looks
much larger. He is something that is eternal, and this has to do
with weather and wind and rain. He emanates strength.

I tell him that I find it all rather difficult to understand. He
looks at me kindly and invites me to come with him. In a
strange way he is very important to me. I feel as though I am
becoming smaller. Then he makes a large, all-embracing
gesture and says that this is a place which encompasses
everything. There is a rock and a wood. Water pours down from
the rock and there is a cave in the rock face. The wind is still
blowing. In this place sunlight is very important and I see there
is also a fire. It is only a small place and yet it has everything.
The old man himself is life. When I look at him I understand
why he says he is eternal. Thus everything acquires a meaning.

Then he takes me back again. I notice that I feel confused.
All the small things are big here. I myself have become smaller
than I was before. What he is trying to explain is too big to be
believed in every day. "That is why it is eternal," he says.

The old man says something about the feelings I carry in me.
He tells me that I should move on. It is important for me to have

seen the island. "The one cannot exist without the other having existed," he says. He also makes something clear to me about the feelings I carry within me. "Experiencing what is ahead of you makes sense only when it becomes eternal and goes on existing. You can't escape it. Feelings which you carry within you exist in order that you may get to know them. Then you will know what life is and why it exists." Then he takes me back to the boat.

And His Name Is "Eternal"

Sometimes you say, "I have only an outside and no inside." You notice this especially in your contacts with other people and with animals. You feel nothing. Only when you are with plants are you able to feel something.

Nor do you like it when people waffle about expressing their emotions; when they talk in that vein you suddenly become very cynical. And all that bleating about sweet little lambs in the spring, you have no use for that either. You don't believe in it, and this is your way of keeping a firm hold.

The fair-haired young man went too far. He made it clear that he cared about you but that was quite impossible. Contact, yes, okay, but only with regard to the external things of life and without touching each other. That is why a large part of him had to be buried, and this was probably his inner part.

Yet this is not what you ultimately have in mind, even though you are glad that for the time being you don't need to worry. There seems to be something deliberate about this whole story. Why did it all have to happen in this way? After a moment the trail seems to continue. The young man has vanished but now another, older man appears who sends out strong radiation, and he too starts talking about emotions.

The driving principle in the story now becomes visible: your path leads to a boat and it is immediately clear what you have to do: you have to get into that boat.[3]

Sailing on the water you discover an island and there you meet the old man, who behaves in a reserved but at the same time impressive way. There is a mysterious haze around him, as if he knew what is behind everything—perhaps in this case I should say what is inside everything. His name is Eternal, and the first thing he does is show you his tiny island. This proves to be meaningful, because, although it is a very small island, everything is present on it. Nothing has been forgotten. Even when things die away, they can still re-emerge in some way or other, as is the case with the inner side of the young man, or so we must hope.

You don't need to believe in this every day, because the world he is talking about goes on revolving for ever and ever. So what is the gist of his remarks? He is saying something about your emotions. It seems as if your emotions don't exist any longer, but he claims that they are still present. They are always present and your task is to get to know them. The events in your life and perhaps also in these imaginations are intended to make you get to know life.

The Village with the Shadows

I am on a voyage in a space ship. Its shape resembles that of a spinning top. We are about to land. It is pitch-dark, as if we were entering a cave.

Inside the cave there are corridors, crisscrossed this way and that, as in a labyrinth. We land on water, and I am floating. The space ship has changed into a cage which lies on the water. We arrive at a place where it is lighter. It is the open sea. The cage remains near the shore. After a time I am washed up on the beach, where I see the most peculiar beings walking around. They are robots with one, two, and three eyes. The robots take me with them to the village which is not far away from there. There is a village square with roadside cafés and at one of these I sit down.

I am sitting at a table with a few other people. They ask me where I have come from. I don't know the answer to that. I say I have just been washed up on the shore and that I don't really know how I got there and even less where I have come from. Then they ask me who I am. When I look at myself I see a whole lot of loose faces, without any connection between them. I find this very confusing. I can't make head or tail of it. Nor am I able to answer the question. I don't know who I am. Then I ask those people with whom I am sitting what kind of a village this is. They say this village is well known because shadows are collected here. They wash up on the beach and sometimes people come here to fetch their shadows back.

And sure enough, when I look around I see people walking around with their shadows. I can see my shadow as well. I recognize it at once. This shadow of mine has to do with my feelings. To my question whether I can get my shadow back, they say that I cannot get it back just yet. I will have to wait till later.

Then the spinning top comes flying along once more. I have to get in again. The shadows that have not yet been collected are all being carefully tidied away. People are very busy with this, they want to clear everything up properly. Then I vanish into space again.

THAT DOOMED FEELING

When we talk to each other between imaginations, I have on occasion heard you speak about feelings. At home, in the evening, when you are on your own, you feel sad and angry, though you don't know about what. In your contact with other people this has all disappeared now. There is only one thing you still have to worry about. People must not come too close to you. And most of all, they must not touch you. They will be allowed to do that only when you have become completely without feeling, you say. So where do you put your feelings?

The story of the village with the shadows provides the beginning of an answer to this question. You might have read C. G. Jung's book about the shadow, but I know you haven't. The word *shadow* simply occurs here, all by itself, and nothing complicated is said about them. People can lose their shadows. Somehow or other it is possible to uncouple that annoying dark fellow-traveler from yourself and leave it behind somewhere.[4] In this strange village you see people walking around with their shadows and you even see your own. It has something to do with your feelings, you say. It would seem, then, that you have begun to make very negative judgments about your feelings. It is always difficult to face up to these negative aspects, but you have now detached yourself completely from your shadow and you have gone off without it. What can have happened, that you found it necessary to doom your feelings so totally? You don't know and I don't know either. We can find out the answer only when you are able to meet your shadow again and pluck up enough courage to confront it. The beginning is there: you have caught a glimpse of your shadow.

At this moment you know only that your main difficulties lie in your contacts with men, and therefore also with your father, and that in order to be on the safe side you have continued your journey with regard only to the external. When, down there in the village, you have to answer the question of who you are, you have no answer. You can see nothing but separate faces. Sometimes you put on one face and then again another, just as it happens or as is required.

If you are to get your shadow back, you will have to wait until the developments have progressed sufficiently. I don't suppose you like to hear this, but it is probably said with good reason. Facing up to those condemned feelings is no small matter. It will require a great deal of courage and strength, and it looks as if the first condition is the creation of a safe climate.

A Strange Fisherman

I am in a tunnel and I see two headlights in the distance. There is a great deal of noise which is coming nearer. It is a train. The tunnel in which I am is very narrow. I am hit and I have a feeling as though half of me is ripped away. I notice that my outline has gone. This is a bewildering feeling but at the same time light. I have a feeling as though I have lost something, but I don't want it back either. It is as if I am closer to myself like this. I am aware that I am walking. It is still very strange. As if I have lost control to some extent.

Outside the tunnel there is a proper path leading between the mountains. A small cart is standing by the side. It is quiet here. There are some animals: a hedgehog and a few rabbits. A white rabbit is sitting in front of me and looks at me. He is very reassuring and soft. I ask him where I am supposed to go. He points at the cart and indicates that I am allowed to use it. A few more rabbits come along to set the cart in motion. It runs on rails. As soon as we have started to move the rabbits jump off. Now I ride on alone.

Down below, someone is fishing in a narrow stream. He walks to the rails and is able to stop the cart. He is obviously there in order to meet me. Now that I have arrived he goes back to the water. He does something very strange. He is not catching any fish. What he catches appear to be icicles. They are of different shapes. He already has a whole pile lying beside him. He does not seem to notice that the ice on the bank is melting. How pointless this is.

Then the fisherman begins to talk to me. He explains that there is nothing pointless about it. He simply fishes up whatever does not belong in the stream. When the ice has melted it is allowed to flow back into the stream again.

He also shows me that there are nets in the water and that therefore a wall of icicles has been formed. I don't understand why he is fishing only those few out of the water. He explains that by picking out the heaviest ones he is making a breakthrough possible. Now I myself go further down the bank. I look at the stream for a while and then I see exactly what he means. The sun shines through the water here, and you can see colors that penetrate deep down into the water. Higher up the stream this was different. The ice acted as a mirror up there, reflecting all the light.

In this way warmth can also penetrate into the water.

The banks are covered with greenery and I see trees standing along the water's edge.

THE COOL FACADE

You've come back for another session. Sometimes I wonder why you do. The concrete problems for which you come are still there, the same as ever and it does not look as if anything is being done about them.

So far you have been told only that your feelings will come back, but that won't help you much with getting through the week. At the same time we must remember that when your feelings do come back, quite a few of those concrete problems will have been solved at the same time. Even so, it seems to me that what you have gained so far doesn't amount to very much.

Let us have another look at the images, to see whether perhaps any hope can be derived from them. An accident happened to you, down there in that railroad tunnel. Is there any glimmer of good luck in that? Your exterior has been ripped away. What do you have left? It is certainly true that people can still get ahead who have nothing at all. In any case, you don't mind in the least having lost your exterior. You'd rather be without than with. It wasn't of much use to you anyway, was it. From the outside you seem big and strong. No one would ever guess you were troubled by some huge life-size problem. Now that this accident has happened to your exterior you will have to realize that this situation will change. People will notice something about you now. They will probably be aware that there is something the matter with you. You yourself will notice it too. You will discover that you are walking by yourself and that you are getting closer to yourself. This will probably mean that you are also going to get closer to others.

How should we imagine this, if your cool facade is taken away from you? The white rabbit will show you what it is like. He has put you on the track of that cunning fisherman. It is really too crazy for words. A fisherman fishing for icicles, what on earth are you to make of that! He tells you something about a breakthrough that is being made possible. It will allow the water to flow through more easily.

You yourself discover yet another effect. The water is acquiring more color and the colors can penetrate deeper into the water. If we could now for a moment assume that colors are rather like feelings, then this might seem to be a small step in the right direction.

In this way your life might acquire more warmth. Stranger still, this must already be happening. Yet you have noticed that there are lots more icicles still under the water, and the fisherman is acting cautiously. He does not pull everything out of the water at once. And then there is a net as well, holding all the ice back. Do you know the icicles in your daily life, and do you know how they hold back the sunlight so that it is refracted from the surface of the water?

The Castle That Keeps Something Imprisoned

In the distance is a point to which I am being drawn. I am standing in the middle of a yellow landscape, very ripe and very round. It is an area of round hills and the trees are also standing in semicircles, with their crowns bending toward the earth. All the colors I see are shades of yellow, even the streets and the houses, and yet it is not sunny.

I walk down a path. In the distance lies a village. It is a very gentle landscape. The houses of the village look like those in a picture by Anton Pieck. Every house has something different about it, a water butt or some kind of special signboard. There are people that look like dolls. They are small and fat and round. It is as if they are looking at me, as if I am being overtaken. I walk through the village and turn into a path that leads upward. It leads up a hill with a castle on it. Everything about the castle is round too, including the turrets.

All the time I am being sucked back to the village. The wind moves the signboards which show me the way back to the inn. The door of the inn is open and I enter. Everything inside is made of wood. I take a seat by the bar. There is another person sitting beside me. It is a young man wearing some kind of uniform. I ask him why I am here. All the time I hear something about a task. It has something to do with the castle. The young man speaks in images. I see a kind of oven. People are waiting for me. There are also two horses. The story isn't very clear to me. There is something which is being held imprisoned here, that is all I can make out. And it also has something to do with that yellow color that everything has, even though there is no sun. There is something very dark in the castle, which is stopping everything.

Outside, the horses are drinking from a trough. Now I am riding one of these horses. The young man is on the other horse. He is riding in front. We are going in the direction of the castle. The closer we get to it, the colder the air becomes. A wall has been built around the castle, with pointed bits of glass all along the top. The horse I am riding is a dark one. Both animals are restless. I know there is something that has to be released. We dismount and continue on foot. Inside the castle, we can hear the sounds of a party. Everywhere in the grounds there are small black figures to be seen. They are covered in black cloth with holes for the eyes.

I know I must get away from here fast. They are waiting for me in the castle.

I must hurry, before they find out what has happened. I am given a horse to ride. When I am already a long way off, I see the roof of the castle opening up. A big flock of black birds comes swarming out of it, in my direction. I must try to get to the forest. We are going very fast. The horse stumbles and I start running. When I reach the forest the birds have just missed me. There is a frontier which they cannot cross. In the forest

there is one more yellow tree, pointing toward the ground. I go
to that tree to sit down and rest.

Weeks have gone by since I was at the castle. I want to try to
find it again.

The landscape in which I am now is white with snow. The
snow makes a crunchy sound under my feet. The village is still
there, but this time I enter it from a different direction. There is
a thick blanket of snow on everything and it is very quiet. In
some of the houses there is light. Many houses have their
shutters closed. The snow lies banked up high against the
doors. It is difficult to recognize the shapes of things. The inn is
still there. Its doorstep has been swept clean. There are lots of
people inside. It is warm in there and a big fire is burning in the
hearth. The people are sitting in a circle around the fire. There
is something odd about the sound. A meeting is in progress but
I cannot understand a word of what is being said. The boy is
there too. He is sitting opposite me and has recognized me.
There is something friendly about him. I wait till the meeting is
over and then I ask him what has happened to the village.

He speaks in images again. Something is wrong with the
castle. The castle does not fit in with the village. There is
something black inside it which holds back the water that
would normally flow into the stream. It is a long story. The
villagers have just been discussing ways in which the castle
could be removed. Efforts have already been made, but because
there is ice all around it they have not been able to set fire to it.
And besides, it never occurred to them that the trouble was not
really the castle itself but what was inside it. The boy and I have
both seen people in it. Perhaps it would be possible for me to go
to the castle, since I was expected there. That is why I am
probably the only person who could knock at the door there.
But I want all these people here to come with me and hide in
the grounds around the castle. Then I won't feel so alone. They
are frightened, I gather. I am angry. It isn't fair what goes on
between the castle and the village. The villagers have to pay for

everything. The castle has complete control over them. They have nowhere to turn any more.

On the way they tell me what goes on up there. When I enter I come upon a large number of figures in black standing in a circle. They try to touch me. I don't want them to touch me. I am very angry because of what they are doing to the village and I start kicking and lashing out.

What I do is not enough, there are too many of them. I defend myself on all sides but I cannot prevent them from touching me. I open my eyes and give them a withering look. That helps, it makes them frightened. I am extremely angry with them. Now that they are shrinking back, I look for the exit. I can reach it without hindrance. Outside, the people are waiting for me. They surround me and take me back to the village. There they look after me. I have become very cold. Blankets are being fetched and the fire is stoked up higher. They have put me on a bench by the window. When I look out I can see the castle. I can see it, but something is happening to it. It is caving in, completely. Only some of the foundations remain.

The Wicked Plan Fails

The yellow landscape in which you are walking is at the same time friendly and strange. Everything is round and gentle, but how can everything be yellow when there is no sun? Meanwhile you have found out how important the sun is. It makes it easier for you to see through the surface of the water. It allows color and feeling to enter into your life. What is going on here? Have all the colors disappeared?

You know from experience in your daily life that it doesn't take much for the whole business to be stuck fast again. A firm approach appeals to you. No messing about. All that pussyfooting, can't it ever stop? Of course it can stop, but the price would be high. You would have to take yourself firmly in hand. Your problem seems to be that you would like to have feelings but that you are at the same time afraid of them. This dilemma causes a great deal of tension. And then you have to fight all the harder to get rid of the tension.

When we enter the village we see some of that fight. You set off for the castle at once. Do you think that is where you most belong? You are being pulled; there is another part of you which does not agree, does not agree with the fact that you choose sides without due thought. You are sent back to the café and there it is explained to you that a dark power rules in the castle, holding something imprisoned which is badly needed by the village and the area surrounding it.

During the conversation it is as if you are gradually being persuaded. The young man introduces the notion that something has to be released and that he needs you to carry out this task. You are expected at the castle and he clearly thinks it would be a good idea to use this as the starting point for the rescue plan. He has already prepared two horses, and then you find yourself in a strangely ambiguous position. You could enter the castle, because you have been invited. You could approach the cordon of black figures around the castle, because you feel that the idea of guard duty suits you. But there is also something exciting in the wicked plan of the young man. To open a window, while a party is in full swing inside. This sort of thing has been done before.

How is it that you have confidence in this young man? Are you quite sure he will offer you enough protection if anything goes wrong? You have probably dismissed the fisherman's warning a little too lightheartedly. He was not in favor of taking down the entire barrier in one go. Take it easy, that was his motto. It is not surprising that the abrupt pulling open of the window gives you quite a big fright, and you are forced to take flight. You are right, you have become a wiser person. The castle is in control of something vital. Vital not only to the villagers but also to you. All feelings are imprisoned in the castle and are being closely guarded. Letting them go by opening a window is not sufficient to free them properly. You will have to strike back at the frightening dark force of the black birds, which you have escaped only by a hair's breadth.

It was this moment in the story that became a central point in your struggle to conquer your difficulties. While in the imagination the experience of being pursued was not exactly pleasant, you had a far worse time of it in the evening after, at home. After hours of torment you came to the conclusion that the images really did have an influence on your life. On the one hand, their influence was bad, because you were frightened out of your wits. On the other hand, it was also a favorable influence. At the next session, to my utter amazement, you wanted to go back to that village and that castle. If that was the place where you were stuck, you wanted to go right back and sort things out.

The next sequence of imaginations shows how you were able to make this coolheaded decision. When you returned to the village, everything was completely frozen over. So that was your reaction to those anxious hours. Everything that had been stirred up there was stuck fast in the ice. Your feelings were further away than ever. A strategy for survival had begun inside you, to maintain life through the winter of famine until the siege would end.

When in that village you are given another chance to talk to the young man, it becomes clear to you that an age-old battle is being fought here. The castle has the power to block the flow of water and the villagers try to fight this by threatening the castle with fire. It is a fight between fire and water.[5] When you have taken stock of the situation it is clear to you: the castle holds the highest trump cards. There are not many fires left in the village.

And then a decision is made which will not be reconsidered: you choose sides once and for all. Stranger still, you not only take your stand on the side of the villagers, but you even take charge. To begin with, this means you have to become a spy. Before the fight can be fought, more and better information is needed. The enterprise is partly an innocent one; after all, you are responding to an invitation and this must imply that you are welcome there.

You are partly aware of the danger, for you know about all those black birds. It is as if the villagers sense what a courageous enterprise this is. They decide to accompany you on your mission, all of them together. For the time being this is no more than moral support. They are too afraid to enter the castle with you.

Your unsuspecting trust proves to have been unjustified. As soon as you enter the castle, the black force that reigns there comes bearing down on you with its full weight. It is a hopeless struggle, no doubt about that. And yet something happens. On your way to the castle, a tremendous feeling of anger had risen in you. You were particularly outraged at the unjust exploitation of the villagers. This anger is precisely what is now so useful to you in your fight against the black figures. They are trying shamelessly to break through your taboo by touching you. During this imagination it was clear from your expression that you were trying to keep those evildoers away from you by kicking and hitting. You succeeded only in part and you had to flee once again. Icy cold and chilled to the bone you emerge from the ice palace and are welcomed by the villagers. In these grim circumstances you are able to receive a little bit of warmth, which is in itself something of a miracle, considering that nothing is more threatening to you than warmth. Yet you succeed in absorbing a very small amount of it.

The parallels with your daily life become more numerous. It is impossible to say what kind of relationship really exists between the events in the imaginations and what you experience in real life. There is no simple causal relationship. That is why I speak of parallels, because at this time you are beginning to mention things like the fact that you sometimes burst out angrily when something happened at work that you didn't like. And you tell me also that you are now finding it almost impossible to deny that there are people who really care about you. Until that moment you had regarded every positive approach as belonging to the world of mere polite gestures that had no true inner content or motive.

It is still only a crack in the ice and a tiny chink in the wall:

there are things that can no longer be denied. Neither the influence of the images nor the influence of an inner reality, as expressed by the behavior of the people, can be disputed any longer.

In the images there is a strange relation between good and evil. There is no clear either-or. Earlier on, the little black figures under the water already said they had your well-being at heart, and now they are driving you into the arms of these villagers. It seems that in spite of your failure in the struggle a victory has been gained nevertheless. The castle falls down, but whether this can be seen as a true victory will have to become clear in what follows next.

The Situation Worsens Visibly

When I return to the café I find the place in chaos. There is no one about. The furniture is broken. I can hear some sounds, though. Then an elderly man comes in, looking dejected. To my question as to what has happened here, I am once again shown the answer in images: many people have died, but a few are still alive. The café had become too big for use. All the woodwork is now being chopped up for firewood. I follow him to a smaller room. It is chock-a-block with people all sitting about doing nothing. They look defeated. I try to make it clear to them that it is stupid, the way they are behaving, but they don't listen and they don't look at me. Then a few more people enter, wearing thick clothing. It is becoming quite unbearable in here. I want them to leave the door open, we ought to get some movement in the place. I fetch some snow from outside and throw it on the fire. This soon makes it cooler. Then at last a few people go out. I want all of them to go outside but they don't move. I daren't touch them either, but I want them to get out. Then I open the windows as well. That helps.

The rest I do with my eyes. They notice this, because they get angry. I have a feeling that I am stronger than they are. But they keep sitting together in a huddle and I want them to start tidying up the café and the village. And after that the people who have been snowed in must be freed as well. And fires have to be lit in order to melt the snow. I am angry because all this time they have been doing nothing. Things are doing a little bit better now, but I keep having to watch these people, or they stop working again. Their faces are beginning to have more expression. And it seems as if I can hear music. They are becoming more alive again. I know I have to remain angry, though, if anything is to be changed here. For the moment they are not allowed back in the café. First all the work has to be finished. Good, now I don't want to look at them any more for a while.

The next time it is a dark day. I walk around the square where there are still banks of snow. A good deal of work has been done, I can see that, but at this moment no one is in sight. All the tools lie scattered around.

In the café there are people. They are wounded and covered in blisters. A first aid post has been set up. They all look very miserable. There has been an attack by birds, they tell me. A great flock of them swooped down on the village.

I look out the window. It seems as if the castle is there again. I feel that I am afraid, now that the castle has come back. The people have noticed it too, the castle has risen from its ruins. This is most disheartening. For the moment nothing much can be done, they say, because they have to regain their strength first. They are also worried that they will not manage to get through the winter. The enemy is too powerful and as so little success has been achieved, everybody is beginning to lose heart. I cannot stand it any longer and I begin to cry. It is as if everyone is laughing at me.

Then I hear them say that contact has been made with the castle. Up there, they are planning to maintain our state of exhaustion. Their power has grown. We in the village must think of something that they are not aware of. It must be something that will frighten them. Some kind of recovery must

be achieved here, over which the castle has no power. But I
can't see how that can be done. First of all, there must be a fire
in every home. Outside the village I have noticed plenty of trees,
so we ought to be able to light fires. The people are beginning to
regain a bit of imagination.

As I am in the company of these people I now dare cast a
brief glance at the castle again. It looks horribly triumphant.
But at the same time this might be their weakness. I don't feel
defeated yet. All we need is time to work out a plan.

This time I approach the village by a different route. I find
myself level with the castle. It is still grim winter weather and
this gives me a safe feeling, because it means I can hide behind
the banks of snow. I can look through the windows. There are
lots of glittering instruments inside. There is an industrial air
about the place. Plans are being prepared in there, I notice.
Something is being done with computers, and cameras are
aimed at the village. This allows them to observe all movement
and activity down there. All the data are put into the computer
and this enables them to take action very quickly.

Down in the village I see smoke circling up everywhere. This
causes confusion in the castle: the number of people does not
tally with the number of fires. I hurry back to the village. On
the way, lots of dark blotches come hovering around my head,
which act like electrified wires. When I arrive in the village I
still see the smoke circling up but the people look vacant. They
don't have much wood left. They behave as if all their strength
has gone. I had better go and get some of those little black
figures from my castle. Perhaps I can use them to scare the
people a bit. Indeed I succeed, for they take to their heels at
once. I walk all around the village with those black blotches,
because I want everyone to realize that it is not yet safe here. I
succeed. All the villagers come out of their houses. I show them
the way to the trees, because the fires must be kept burning.

Meanwhile I have made contact with the castle. Confusion
still reigns up there, and has in fact increased. They are

counting on it that down in the village everyone sits waiting
despondently for things to happen. A new confusion has arisen
now, because footprints have been detected all over the place, of
people who have gone to collect wood. The castle is expanding.
This is probably because they are trying to gain more strength.
But they are not aware that I know how it all works. We must
see how we can turn the tide.

One thing is certain, there should be more life in the village.
All the shutters should be taken away from the windows. Then
I show the people in images what the village could look like. In
fact, they should be doing the exact opposite of what they are
doing. Next time I want to see the market square swept clean
and a market being held.

Then I see the boy approaching with whom I opened the
window in the castle earlier on. There is a look of recognition in
his eyes. At last someone who understands me. We decide that
there ought to be sounds and smells. He is able to work with
sound boxes and moreover he knows everybody in the village
and what everyone can do. I also explain to him that there ought
to be far more people. Dolls must be made, so that up there in
the castle there will be even more confusion. It won't be possible
to get everything done at once, but there will come a time when
there won't be any more snow. Then this will be a very fine
village and at the place where the castle is now there will be
something very different. A funfair will appear there, with a
roller coaster and a Big Dipper. And it will be spring, the time
for spring cleaning.

The Iron Lady

This must be a real disappointment to you: the collapse of the
castle has not led to an improvement in the situation in the village. On the contrary, there is famine and people are suffering
pain. Some are dead, others wounded. The castle clearly had an-

other function besides being a symbol of a hostile power. It kept the black force more or less within bounds. Now disaster has struck the village. There are casualties to be mourned.[6]

The military forces of which you have taken charge are now totally demoralized. Your commands are not being followed. There is no longer any possibility of communication. This makes you angry again and you decide to rule with a strong hand. More of the same, that is your motto. You throw out the last little fire. You actually adopt the fighting tactics of the castle. Snow over it. If there is to be more fire, then there will first have to be less. Slowly things begin to liven up a little.

What does all this have to do with you? In our conversations you said that for many years you did all kinds of things in order to draw attention to yourself, so that it would at least seem as if people cared about you. To achieve this end you took extreme measures, like inflicting injuries upon yourself, in order to get a certain amount of attention. It did not have much effect, but it was important as a substitute all the same.

Here in the village you stir up the people to take notice of the injured victims buried under the snow. It seems like fighting against a brick wall. The number of injured is increasing and there is a general air of despondency. The castle has risen again.

The triumph of the castle even seems to have grown. This is a minor error of judgment on the part of the opposite side. They should not have been so proud. You are beginning to get a glimpse of the strategy that is being employed, and then the iron lady inside you stands up. If war has to be waged, you can play your part. The end appears to justify the means. Now that you have seen that those in the castle act in a purely calculating way and observe all the movements in the village, the time has come to use cunning. You partly succeed in doing so, but the villagers remain the weak link in the chain. They are outdone every time.

Your despair must have reached its peak because you now set off to collect arms from near by the castle. Those little black figures of which you yourself were so afraid earlier on, you now use against the people on your own side in order to set them on their

feet again and get them to replenish the stock of firewood. This is
how you deal with yourself too. Crying is no use, give them
the whip.

An Old Acquaintance Returns

I stumble over toadstools. Mist hangs close above the ground.
The toadstools are growing near the stumps of felled trees. I feel
all kinds of obstacles under the snow. The wind comes toward
me. There is a smell of smoke. Now the village comes into view.
Smoke can be seen everywhere. At last the ground becomes
visible in patches among the houses. It is quiet. In the village
square the snow has all been swept to the side. When I enter the
café I see a wheel turning with lots of images on it. I can stop it
turning, and then I realize what is going on: the people are all
busy in a large shed. They have made something that looks like
a railroad engine. There is a great deal of activity. Someone is
standing by the door. It is a man, he is talking animatedly. There
have been many setbacks and there are many casualties, but the
fires have gone on burning all the time. With the engine they
will be able to push the snow aside more easily. For the first
time I see that everybody is really working hard. They have
realized that fire can be used to good purpose, and that it can
have an effect on the castle. I ask them who has managed to
achieve this. It is a young person with a radiant face. It is the
same boy as last time, but I had not seen him so clearly before.
He looks very strong. Now I am walking through the streets. It
is busy. I keep having to step aside. There is something strange
about it all, because the people aren't real. They are merely
painted, to give the appearance that there are many of us.
　　Now I arrive at a house where someone is sick. I can see this
in a double image. There is also a boy, the same one that I met
some months ago at the campsite in the dunes. I see again
before me how I buried him that time and how he himself stood
watching me. Here, too, he is double, as before, for he is

standing by his own sickbed. The boy tries to explain
something to me: "He is no different from what I am myself,"
he says. When I ask whether I can help him we go outside
together. Suddenly I remember what he said at the moment of
his burial. "What is being buried here is only that part of me
that causes a wall to exist between us. From now on you will
always be able to reach me, but you may also go away if you
want, because you can never get rid of me." This has all come
true, I think. I have gone away from him because I could not
bear having him so close by. As we are walking outside together
he explains to me that the villagers must first gain some more
strength before we are able to fight against the castle. Briefly I
see the image of the sick boy in the bed. "This is not a trick,"
he says, "I am alive when you are here and I am sick when you
stay away."

The Masculine Counterpole

Time and again we have seen that the frozen water does not have
a proper counterpart. The little fires in the village were too weak
and too few in number.

You have succeeded in getting people to work, by force and
especially by frightening them, but you also need a certain perspective. It is necessary to develop vision. You need that for yourself. If all you do is constantly exert yourself without any relief,
you can't keep going in the long run. Gradually something like a
vision is born in you. One day the time will come when there is
no longer any snow on the ground. It will be spring then, and
you cannot imagine anything more wonderful than spring time,
with a fairground.

This is what you keep saying both to yourself and to the people,
and at last some progress can be made. The young man, with
whom you opened the window at the castle, has come back. He
represents the lost part of yourself, your male counterpart.[7] Once,
very long ago, you met him as the young man with the fair hair

and now he has come back from somewhere. Or have you come back from somewhere?

Whichever it is, you had lost each other, and much of your trouble was due to this fact. The health-giving equilibrium between the male and female elements had been completely lost. Now that the mechanization in the village has got underway, you wonder who is the mastermind behind it. On inquiry it appears to be a radiant young man.

All kinds of things are changing in you: a vision has developed, you act purposefully, and, perhaps most important of all, you are no longer alone in taking initiatives. The young man does something too. But he can act only under certain conditions. You become aware of this when you stand by his sickbed. When you are in contact with him, he is alive. If you go away from him, he is sick. Of course you don't have a great deal of influence over this. If you did, you would have fixed things long ago. No, there are unconscious causes which so far have prevented you from succeeding, and even now you succeed only partly.

Looking at it superficially, you might say that if the male pole has been lost from sight, it should surely be possible to go on living with only the female pole. But it isn't as simple as that. The young man himself has hinted as much; he is sick when you leave him. But the reverse is true as well; when he leaves the scene you are very sick indeed. Not that you are aware of this every minute of the day, but as soon as you are on your own for a moment or when, in some personal contact, you have to reveal yourself, you are unable to do what other women can do. The female pole then proves to be impaired as well.

A Three-Cornered Game of Checkers

The view is immense. I am standing with my back to a wood. There is a frontier here. Before me lies a vast winter landscape, with the village in the middle. Behind me, in the wood, the

climate is quite different. There are not many leaves on the
trees, but there is no longer any snow on the ground. In the sky
the clouds also run up against a frontier. Along a certain
invisible line they turn back again. It gives me a feeling of
observing something which is finite.

For the first time some of the stores are open in the village. I
go to the café. Inside, some people are playing a game. There
are three of them, all men, playing at a three-cornered board
with checkers on it. I don't know this game. It is very quiet in
here. I want to go outside again, because something isn't right.
Certain things are missing. Although there are some people in
the street, none of them carry any shopping with them.

In the shed there is a lot of noise. There are large boards on
the wall on which rows of names are written with crosses after
them. Behind a table five people are filling out forms. They are
writing up work schedules for teams of workers. A great deal
has been done, I hear, and yet the village is in a bad state.
Instead of apathy there is now activity but nothing else. There is
a certain amount of life, but there is less and less to eat.

Meanwhile I have gone in search of the young man, but he is
nowhere to be found in the village. I keep seeing an image of a
road behind the castle. I see the boy sitting there. Something
has happened to him. He seems to be wounded. And there is
something around him which makes it impossible for me to get
to him. The castle has locked him inside an invisible ball. A big
black monster with three legs has captured him and thrown him
by the side of the road. When I come close to the ball I feel fear.
I must go and fetch help. I put a glove near him and go back to
the village to get assistance. There I see the three men from the
café. They are on their way to the boy but they are carrying
their checkerboard with them. We have to be quick, because
dark clouds are gathering behind the castle. Then I see that the
checkerboard has been put down in front of the boy. The three
men take each other by the hand, thus forming another triangle.
The legs of the two triangles intersect, forming a star. In a
strange way there is now a central point and the boy is exactly at

that point. Now something has snapped and I can hear thunder and wind. The boy has come out of the ball. I pick up the glove and I know that we must hurry away from here. It is hailing ice cubes now, so that the castle is no longer to be seen. The three men are standing around us and form a cupola in which we sit. They have not survived. When we arrive at the village I ask everyone to come out. I know that those three men want to be burned. They are lying in a place where people have been burned previously. I don't know why, but I want to watch the burning. There is an enormous funeral pyre, on which the three men are lying. I know that what happens here is good. But it is terrible to see. When the fire goes down, everybody turns round. The boy has stayed with me. I gather he wanted to go to the castle, but an attack was made on him. If this had not happened he would have slowly suffocated. Now it is getting dark. I have decided to stay the night here.

When I wake up I look out through a window. Icicles are hanging from the eaves. Indoors there are piles of logs. The place I am in looks like some sort of shed.

Outside, the weather is gray, and visibility is poor. When I open the door I am at once in the village square. I feel the cold wind. Yet it does not seem as if much has changed. Small groups of people are standing about. Now I see that the people have formed a long line, ending at the place where the three men were burned, at the foot of the castle. The line begins by the shed and logs are being passed from hand to hand. A very tall pyre has been built. It is not likely that much of this can be seen from the castle, because visibility is so poor. It is still very early in the morning.

The people seem to be walking in a particular way. They are resolute and, unlike other times, they behave as if they know exactly what they are doing. Nothing is said and it seems as if I am the person who has given instructions for all this. They are busy collecting the last few logs. There is a plan, because they all take up their position in a semicircle around the castle, with their backs to the pyre. When the pyre is lit there is no road back any more. I know there are plans for an attack. They want a sign from me.

Then suddenly everything happens very quickly. Doors are pushed in. The whole crowd of people storms into the castle. It is dark in there and something black is moving about. It consists of long strands that come from all over the place. It skims over the floor and all the people are getting buried underneath. It is very sticky. It is as strong as we are. They cannot win and neither can we. I don't understand at all what is going on. I am standing at the center. The black thing is now inside the people. Something has happened to the castle. It is empty and yet it is not. It is as if a fusion has taken place. The people are there and so is the blackness. I can see myself also, with lots of little black dots sticking out of me. It is as if some part of them is now inside me. Part of the castle is now in me. It feels as if it isn't quite in the right place yet. Everything billows and moves.

From inside the castle I can look out through a window, across the village. The fire is burning the top layer of earth. The ground sinks and the village disappears into the depths of the earth. From underneath the castle a new layer of earth begins to pour out over the valley. It seems to be fertile soil, in which much can grow. New houses rise out of the ground. The village is being formed anew.

On the other side of the village I see someone waving. It is the boy with the fair hair, calling out to me. There is a path all around the village, so I can go to him. I feel emotion welling up inside me. I know he is waiting for me. For the first time I know that all this is really about me. So many people have always said this to me but I could never feel it. Now I know I do not have to go on alone any further.

Together we sit on the top of the hill and look out over the village. The castle is still there, but the colors have changed. In its present state, the castle fits in better with the village. The boy has also changed. He seems to have grown older. He tells me something in images. He shows me that he has always been here, but that there were things which I had to do alone.

Otherwise it would not have been possible for me to see him. Now I feel more strongly that he is able to protect me.

THE LANDSLIDE

To bring the male and females poles together again is a difficult task, if in the course of time they have become so totally disconnected as in your case. In the unconscious part of your Self the two are fighting a war of life and death. When that happens it is no longer possible to bring about an encounter without a great deal of effort.

In your contacts with people, a wall has arisen which at the same time protects and divides you from others, and this is especially the case in your contacts with men. Yet you would very much like to have an encounter. In practice, therefore, you make desperate attempts to bring one about. By adopting a purely external, not felt, pattern of behavior, you have managed to keep up appearances for a long time. But it has gradually become impossible to maintain the illusion as far as boyfriends are concerned. You are still capable of making love or something approaching it, but afterward a complicated cleansing ritual always has to be performed. Who touches pitch will be defiled by it, and to you men are pitch. You don't think this consciously, for you would love to be happy like other women. Unconsciously though, men are pitch, and here you have the black force, which plays such a dominant part in the bitter struggle of water and fire.

In the reality of your life, sexual contact has become a total failure. One disappointment has followed another and yet you keep fighting to win through. The measures you have to take after each encounter become ever more rigorous. In the end it has come to the point that even after an ordinary visit from your father you have to clean the whole house, or at any rate all the places where he may have been, because otherwise you can no longer feel safe.

In order to put an end to this situation a special operation is necessary. It is as though deliberately some very abstract figurations are being used for this. It involves the use of triangles by means of which a perfect example of a ritual is enacted. You have witnessed it all from close by, but the true significance you could understand only in retrospect, and not until much later. In fact, I think you would have put a stop to it if you had been able to see through it at the time. The preparations for the ritual were already contained in your encounters with the young man in the village. He is slightly less of a stranger to you than all the other people there. At least he understands you and he is a competent deputy when you yourself are absent for a week or so. From time to time he even takes the initiative himself.

On this occasion he lies wounded by the side of the road leading to the castle. Some time ago you also found him injured, somewhere in a valley in the dunes. You tried to help him then, but it was not possible. Now you make a similar attempt. More even than before it is important to you that he should continue fighting together with you. However, once again it seems as if you cannot help him. There is a glass dome between you and it looks as if he won't live much longer. In great haste you rush off to fetch help, which you find in the form of three men. Impossible to imagine anything more masculine. Fortunately your attention is distracted by the mysterious game of checkers. It is as though the three men don't take their task too seriously. They briefly lend a hand and then carry on playing checkers.

The intermingling of the two triangles into a six-pointed star is a symbolic event, one that people in ancient times had learned to interpret as representing the coming together of opposites, in particular of water and fire, and also of male and female.[8] These are exactly the opposites that are causing you so much trouble.

If it is at all possible to understand these things, then this is not in itself the most important thing that is being asked of you here. What matters most is that you experience and undergo the events, so that certain shifts can then take place within you, and the interminable struggle can at last come to an end. This has indeed happened, you have experienced the ritual with an intensity that caused your whole body to convulse and tremble. The symbolic intermingling of the two triangles gave the impulse to a powerful shock wave. Besides, the whole entourage was also guaranteed to make a tremendous impression on you.

First of all there was the black three-legged monster. This is too remarkable to escape your attention. Derived from the number three, which is known to be a masculine number, this monster may be assumed to represent the terrifying appearance of the male element in the unconscious part of your Self. The figure itself is threatening and menacing, and the glass dome in which the young man is imprisoned has also acquired a frightening character. In addition there are the dark sky, thunder and flashes of lightning, and finally the shower of ice cubes raining down on the heads of the three men.

The formation of the six-pointed star is followed by a cleansing operation, similar to those you perform in your own life, except in this case they do not involve the use of water. Fire is used here.[9] In some mysterious way you have discovered the last wish of these men, and you respect this wish. It has cost you an effort. You knew it was good, but it was also a terrible experience. The knowledge that an action has a purifying effect is small comfort at such a time. Of course it is true that these men have only themselves to blame. They belong to the villagers' forces. By venturing so near the castle and moreover by trying to release a prisoner there, they have brought their fate upon themselves. On the other hand they seem to be no more than checkers in a game. They are defeated.

How is this ritual of cleansing by fire to be interpreted? What is the stain they are being cleansed of? Is it the stain of having chosen sides in the war? These questions remain unanswered. We cannot be sure but in some way or other they are exonerated. And if the intermingling of the triangles was intended to signify that at last the end of the struggle is in sight, then this would be perfectly plausible. In that case they have made an essential contribution to the conclusion of peace. Whether something of this sort is indeed the fact we can infer only from the form in which they will next reappear. It is certain that they will reappear. In this psychological world no energy is ever lost. If we now return to the story, we see that the next morning there is still no question of peace. On the contrary, the fire at the place of sacrifice is being stoked up afresh and the decisive battle is about to begin. All you know is that it will be a bitter fight.

Inside the castle you find out about that black pitch-like substance, but what happens next is something very different from what you had expected. The other people and you become permeated by the black substance and although it is not immediately in the right place, you do now have the feeling as though it is part of you. There is no longer a contrast, there is instead a certain equilibrium. That which previously made you so anxious and which you therefore kept far away from you has now become resident in you, and has therefore clearly lost its destructive influence on you.

Through the windows, the positive effect of the process of integration can also be perceived outside the castle. A landslide is taking place there, which will make new growth possible.

And on the other side of the village, like a true counterpole, you see the young man. The meeting between you is touching. Very briefly you feel what you have so often heard others say, that there is such a thing as feeling safe and protected. You now feel that everything is happening for your benefit.

And although the black substance is not yet in the right place, you have nonetheless already experienced a kind of parallel in your daily life. For the first time ever you had a feeling of safety when a friend put his arm around you. The first step has been taken.

The Eternal One with the Three Swans

I am walking along rails in the direction of a wood with very thick trees. There is not much of a path. The trees are bare and the branches are completely entangled with each other. I arrive at a wide path where I see an animal standing. It's very large—a

kind of elephant but with long black hair. It has been waiting
for me.

When I come closer, it stamps on the ground and in doing so
makes the whole scene move. Then it utters a roar, so that a
shiver goes through the wood. A circle is formed which locks
me in. I can no longer see what is happening behind the trees.
Then I walk up to the animal. It takes a few steps backward and
turns. Black snakes twist around the branches above my head. I
follow the large elephant.

We arrive at a small lake. There is another snake there, which
keeps diving under the water. I know that very soon the colors
will change. Then I see three white swans appear. They carry a
large leaf with them. They wait quietly until I sit down on the
leaf. Then the water begins to move. It starts to rain and the
wind gets up. I am carried away on the leaf.

All around me there is only water now, very rough. The three
swans are swimming around me. There is now a very dense
wall of water. Then the dark outline of a boat looms up. The
swans take me to the boat. There is someone on board. It is the
old man from the island where I once went. He helps me on
board and looks at me with great understanding. I tell him I no
longer know where I am. He points around him at the world
which is always there. Where he is everything is eternal. Now
he shows me the castle in images. As with a dolls' house, he
opens up the front. The interior that is revealed is very warm.
He explains that there is plenty of time to refurbish and
rearrange all the rooms of the castle, one by one. And from now
on colors should not be removed from it but added. There is as
yet no point in opening the windows, as long as the interior is
still so empty.

I tell him I don't understand it, and also that I still don't
know where I am.

He says that all this has no time and no space, because it is
eternal. And he himself is called the Eternal One. He will take
me back to the castle. The exterior looks chilly and cold. He

explains that many rooms are still unheated and locked. It is raining again.

THE WORLD THAT IS ALWAYS THERE

After the upsetting events connected with the cremation of the three men and the dramatic changes that have occurred in the situation of the village and the castle, you have slightly lost your bearings. Wasn't it all about a war then? Wasn't that what you always thought? And now suddenly it has all come to an end! The fighting parties have merged with each other. The contradictions have been canceled out. What next? What is being asked of you, now that no more spying activities are required and no more ruses have to be invented?

What is the meaning of this revolution? The people don't want to go back to the village, they feel safe in the castle and so do you. For a moment there is a vacuum, you have no idea what is to be done next.

However, this is a lull before a storm. Against an impressive backdrop of dark trees in which countless snakes are wriggling above your head there stands, as a symbol of strength and solidity, the black mammoth. The wood and everything in it obeys his command, and the majestic beast blazes a trail for you to the waterside. Three swans are waiting for you or, if we may say so, the three men who previously fulfilled a mediating role are waiting for you, but now in a different guise.[10] Through rain and wind they carry you across the choppy waters to the boat in which you rejoin the Eternal One. Once again you are in the world which is always there. It is the world in which villages vanish into the ground and rise again from it renewed, where men change into swans and rituals with triangles bring about a reversal of destiny.

We, who are so accustomed to determining the time and place of everything, find it difficult to get used to the fact that our world also has a reverse side. Or perhaps it would be better to say that our inner world takes account of a different time. In that time no wars need to be won, for in the struggle against yourself you are the victim and there is no victor. The conflicts are solved from within and at a given moment it will become clear to you how you can contribute your share. What is expected of you now is revealed by the Eternal One himself. He shows you that in the castle there are various rooms that have been cold and dark for a long time. It is up to you to open them and bring warmth to them, and especially to bring more color to the castle. You still have no idea what is inside these rooms, and even less how you might be able to open them.

Don't worry; you can leave this to your unconscious Self. It will make sure that you receive new tasks, and you now know what it is all about.

Back to the Source

There is a sound of falling water. It is the sound of a small stream. The water comes from above. I climb up by the side of the stream. Right at the top, where the stream begins, is a faucet. I notice that it has been turned wide open.

Now I am not far from the castle. The stream runs behind the castle and the village. The people from the village are busy carrying stones. I walk toward the hill of the triangles. A hole has been dug there and it is being filled layer by layer with earth and stones. I ask someone who is standing there what it is going to be. I gather that the water runs through it and that the entire hole acts as a kind of sieve.

Then he explains by means of images what kind of stones these are that they are using. They are tomb stones. The image that comes next is of the graveyard in the village where I was born. I am there now, and I know I am not allowed to be there. At the entrance to the graveyard is a notice and it says something about "unaccompanied children." I hear voices. There are trees and shrubs and there is a wide ditch all around the graveyard.

There is someone behind me. I feel frightened because I am not alone here. And there is no one who can help me. I hide behind a shrub and see someone walking past. If only I am not discovered! A friend of mine calls me. She is very far away. I cannot catch up with her. My legs are too short. I am very small.

Now I am sitting on the swing in the back yard at home, with my back to the house. Upstairs in the house I hear voices. They are talking about school, as usual. I always used to be very frightened there. The voices are very loud and I flee to my room, where I start reading a book. It is a scary book and I get frightened again. I want to get away from here.

It becomes black before my eyes and everything starts to whirl about. When I am able to see clearly again I am at the castle. There is a fire. I am looking at the fire. There is a lot of noise as well. I can't hear what is being said, but there are still very loud voices. I see my parents, as they were then. They are having a terrible argument. There is a war of words between them. I stay near the fire.

A moment later the boy with the fair hair has joined me.

"It's all right," he says.

I don't need to look at the fire any longer.

He shows me the hole in the hill and says everything will be all right. I can stay here now. Everything has become quiet and the fire is simply fire.

THE PAST RETURNS

This is the beginning: right at the top of the stream a faucet has been turned on.[11] Up to now everything was symbolic. We could only guess what it was all about. An internal conflict has been solved, that much we know. But what was the conflict about? And who were the parties? We don't know, at least not yet.

In the imagination we deal with next, you return to the source and we can say that in doing so you return to the past. Little by little you will re-experience that which is the cause of all the anxiety existing in your present life. Considering that up until now everything has been progressing very methodically, we may perhaps assume that there is a good reason why you have not had this experience long ago. It is as if the unconscious Self has dared to confront the cause of the conflict and to relive the experience, only now that enough stability and trust have been built up for this to be bearable. Reliving an experience is in itself pointless; an entirely new solution will have to be found as well, and that will demand a great deal of strength of you.

A purification plant is being constructed, for which strange building bricks are used. By means of this installation a link is cast back to a very distant past, when as a little girl you accidentally found yourself in a graveyard, where you were not allowed to be. Uh-oh, where can you go if anyone sees you? Behind that bush is best, because there are ditches all around.

When you get home you sit down on the swing to catch your breath. But no. Behind your back a barrage of loud voices breaks loose and you want to make sure you do nothing that might make the conflict worse. You run upstairs and start reading scary books so that later you will be able to say that you are so frightened because of the things you have just been reading about.

At those moments when there were no books to which you could attribute your fears, there were insects and when there were no insects you could see still more terrifying animals in your imagination. Little by little, reality became distorted and after some time no one was able to understand any longer what was the matter with you. You yourself began to believe more and more firmly that your fears were totally absurd. Reliving this experience is not pleasant. The fears come back in their full intensity, but fortunately the castle and the boy with the fair hair are usually there, and then you can recover your breath.

The Tree of Life

I am walking along a sandy track with blackberry bushes on either side. It is very quiet here, dusk is beginning to fall. It has been a warm day. Everything seems to be waiting for a shower

of rain. I see flashes of lightning in the distance. The cows are
huddling close together in the field. I am standing behind the
village where I was born, where one tree sticks out above
everything, near my home. Behind the roof of the house you can
see the castle.

Suddenly there is a great shock. The tree splits in half. It has
been struck by lightning. The air all around trembles with the
various sounds. One part of the tree lies across the road, the
other half has fallen against the house. I am now by the castle. A
terrace has been built there, and there are three large gulls, each
standing on a stone. When they fly away they each hold a tip of
a sheet, a square white street, which is then spread over the
school and our house. The gulls alight on the fallen tree.

A moment later they have returned to their stones. Close in
front of me I see the tree, lying in two halves. In one place, close
to the roots, the two halves are still joined together. Some of the
roots have remained in the ground.

Dark things are coming out of a hollow in the tree. They
cover the tree. I take hold of the young tips of the roots and
scoop earth over them. I want to forestall the black substance,
before it has covered the whole tree. There is no time to fetch
help. The black stuff is growing and growing and I myself am
now completely covered under it. The new root has been buried
just in time. The black substance can't get at it now. I see the
rest of the tree shriveling up. It becomes very dark around me. I
walk away from the tree and lie down in the water somewhere,
until all the blackness has washed off me.

At the castle a lot of people have assembled. A movie is going
to be shown. The people want to know why all these things are
happening to them. In the movie, fragments from my childhood
are shown, in rapid succession. I am standing at the back of the
screen. I can only half see what is going on. The sound is very
loud and this is unbearable. Lights are flashing. Something
snaps inside my head. Then it is dark.

Everything is silent now. The birds are sitting around me.
There is a very slow movement. A feeling as if I am being
rocked gently until I am calm. There is a very soft light. As if I

were lying in the clouds. The birds have put me here. I no
longer dare look. I am lying curled up, wrapped in a feather
blanket. I still see the birds very faintly.

A TORN EXISTENCE

You still know the facts of many of the scenes that rise to the surface. Only the accompanying feelings have gone. You have even
begun to think that your childhood was a very carefree one. Now
that week after week so many unhappy feelings have been coming up, you know deep down that it wasn't like that. But you
haven't yet gone home, nor have you restored the old representation of the events. How have you managed to make it seem as if it
had all left you stone cold? For some weeks now we have known
that you lived in a torn world: on the one hand you belonged at
your home and school, where your father worked, and on the
other hand you belonged with your friends and with the village,
and in your own mind these two worlds could not be combined.
The constant discipline problems at school made you feel like
sinking into the earth. You wanted to belong to both sides and
not throw in your lot with one camp only. The result was that
you risked not belonging to either side and that was the least
bearable option of all.

The solution to this terrible dilemma is portrayed in the story
of the tree. In reality the tree is still standing up, not split in half.
The story of the tree therefore tells us something about what has
happened to you. One summer evening your life was suddenly
broken in half, with one blow. Not altogether; near the root the
two parts remained joined to each other, so you still knew that it
was possible to live in two different ways, but not both at the
same time. The emergency measure had succeeded: you were
able to go on living in a situation in which it was not possible to
live. Not to have any feelings was the price you had to pay for
belonging, even though you belonged only in part. Your fears
were removed to those moments when you were alone. The old
problem had been solved.

With the new problem you struggled for years. You could mix

with other people only by not fully taking part and keeping them
at a distance. No one was allowed to touch you, for if they did
they would touch the root of your existence, and no new tree had
as yet sprouted from this root. This particular imagination demonstrated that a new tree was being prepared. To this end a risky
operation had to be carried out. Small black figures, which have
so often troubled you in the past, now seem to be aiming for the
tree, which is already so badly damaged. It is now your task to
protect the new shoot, and you know exactly how to do that.
After the cleansing operation the three birds rock you to sleep, as
a sign that all is well.

The Black Phantom

I am at the castle. There are people all around me. It is as if I
can't reach them. They stand in a circle and start walking. Then
they sit down in small groups, each with a separate task. They
are sitting at some distance from each other and try with their
hands to come closer to someone else. Walls arise between them
when they get too close.

I look for someone to talk to. Behind the door I hear voices
and I go toward them. Inside, a movie screen has been set up
and there are pictures and sounds. On the screen I see a path
leading from the castle to a water. The picture tells me where I
have to go. When I look outside I see the path there too.

I have now left the castle behind me, and I am on my way to
the black water. There the ground sinks away under my feet,
and I end up in the dark water. I am touched by things I cannot
see. I think they are hands. The water carries me along, but the
hands do not let me go.

Then it becomes light, and I wash up on a beach near a
village. It is a large village, and the buildings are very tall.
People are standing alongside the road. On either side there is a
line of people whom I recognize from the past. They are people
from the village in which I lived as a child. They know me too.

I have no choice but to pass between the lines. At the end is my father's school, with its windows open. I can only go in one direction, and that is toward the school, but I don't want to go there. The people keep watching me, and they are angry with me because I belong to the school and they are on bad terms with it.

Now I am behind a big tree where they can't see me. As soon as I am out of sight, they begin to disperse. The school stays where it is, and I go to it in order to close the windows.

There is a hole in the wall, and out of it comes an animal. It has many heads and arms. I can't escape. Very slowly it crawls toward me. Help! It is very close to me. I see how it flows away in all directions. Now it has become an ink stain, which disappears under the floor of the school. I want to get away from here. Now I am back at the castle. When I am inside it, there is no one with me. I close the door behind me. I am all right now. It is very quiet here. I feel sad and have only myself. For the moment nothing else is possible.

The room I am in is new. It is completely blue and there is a bed on the floor with lots of pillows. Nothing comes in from outside now. It is quiet and clean here and it is alive. The room is here for me. Here I am safe.

THE CONFRONTATION

The preparations have been very thorough. You have been back to the village of your childhood many times now. It was anticipated that this would make you afraid, because a number of protective measures were taken.

The very first time, for example, all kinds of things were left out of the village. Your house was not there and the school had been taken away. Moreover, all the inhabitants had been removed.

A few times later all the buildings were complete, but the inhabitants were still absent, and now at last the moment has come; everything is here. The whole operation is started off by the inhabitants of the castle. They portray a scene in which they are able to reach each other only up to a certain point. As soon as they seem about to touch each other, walls arise between them.

Now we are coming straight to the point. Who will be boss in your life, that many-headed monster, which is always, everywhere, elusively present? Or will you be boss, because you are stronger than that sly, creeping force? We have seen what happened. As soon as you arrive in the village you are hemmed in on all sides. You can't move sideways or backward. Only one way is still open to you and that is forward. Before you is the school. The windows are open. All the racket and rumpus can therefore be heard by anyone passing by. Blocking your ears will no longer be of any use. The old solutions are no longer sufficient. Not feeling anything does not help. Nor does denying that anything is wrong. A new solution will have to be found, one that is less damaging to you. This is possible, because you are now much bigger than you used to be, and you have been trained for a whole year in dealing with frightening situations.[12]

For a brief instant you still try the old method: if I don't see the people, they don't see me either and will go away all by themselves. But there is no escape. All alone you come face to face with that dreadful black monster and you see. . . . At the moment you think you are going to be beaten, you see that the monster is giving ground. Like an ink stain as large as the classroom he disappears under the floor of the school. You have defeated the monster with your eyes.

The power of the phantom has been broken. You have gone to the limit of your strength. It has been a great strain on your nerves.

As usual there is a little road that cuts through to the castle. If anyone were to meet you now, it would be too much for you. But there is no one to be seen. You are taken straight to a room which you have not seen before. The door locks itself. Not a sound can be heard any more. There is nothing now except the healing, reassuring blue color.[13]

The Talisman

It is hazy around me. Water drips from a rock. Along the side of a small stream runs a path and I follow it.

It is dark there. Very faintly I can see something. It is a cabin and near it stands a tall, strong man, whom I seem to know. We have a conversation without words. He lets me sit on a bench and takes something away from me, which makes me cry. He can take away all the things I am responsible for. Just for this moment I don't need to do anything. I am small. The man quietly goes on working in the garden. He has dug a big hole and puts everything into it that "must" go. It is a crazy sight. Now he gets out a map which is totally crumpled, showing a lot of paths. The castle is on it and there is a path to the water where the village with the shadows lies. Every place I have ever been to is on it. The map is really much larger, for we have only a part of it here. The place with the cabin is on the back. It is not a place like all the others. It is rather like the spot where I met the Eternal One.

There is a broad highway marked on the map. The man shows me that I am standing somewhere on this road, and every place I have ever been to leads to this road. In front of me there are many more paths leading into this road, and so it goes on.

The man gives me a branch with buds, which will probably burst soon. He also gives me a chain with a pendant on which a crossroad can be seen with a circle around it. These are four roads linked with each other by means of the circle. I carry the branch with me and at the moment I put the chain around my neck the cabin and the man have both vanished. In front of me is the castle. There we must wait for the sun. Inside, people are busy. They want to open the windows but it is still too cold outside and as long as the sun does not shine they are busy indoors tidying up. When the castle is ready they can go back to the village. The boy has already gone there. He has been gone for a long time, because he wants to be there when the trees come out of the ground. On the roof of the castle there is a flower pot in which nothing is growing as yet. I notice that the people are looking at the branch I have brought along. I take it up the stairs with me and put it in the flower pot. It stands up straight in the earth.

The castle is now of a lighter color than before, since the

water has begun to flow. I know that near here there is a shed in which seeds can be found. Around the castle everything is still very bare. It is time to start sowing.

Indoors, everyone is still waiting for it to get warm.

THE GOOD OMEN

Too much has been asked of you. Every journey to the village of the past was an ordeal. Your only hope was the castle, which you reached in the end. Sometimes you managed to get there under your own steam, at other times the three birds came to fetch you, but always there came a moment of peace. You were able to trust that your fear would not have the last word. However far you strayed, you always arrived back at the same point and then you were all right again.

This time you started off with reluctance. Was there never going to be an end to all this trouble? Once again you had made preparations for a crusade. How strange then was the experience on this occasion. The crusade did not fit into the sequence. Something pleasant at last. You had to get used to that. Fortunately, the strong man minds his own business. Nothing difficult is being demanded of you. On this one occasion everything is done for you, and all "musts" disappear into the hole in the ground. Then an interim balance sheet is drawn up. You are shown how the imaginations of this year fit into a total plan. To do this, a creased map is produced. Crumpled up in the pocket of a gardener, O heavenly nonchalance, there is the ordinance survey map of the rescue operation which is to enable you to lead an ordinary human life, you, who live two lives at once and are not happy with either. And then you receive presents. A branch with buds ready to blossom: that is promising, and a talisman that no one believes in anymore. But you savor the significance of it: all roads, however much they may look like false trails, are caught in a circle which holds them together. In this way, all the roads are linked with one another. When you put the chain around your neck, there is no need for the strong man to stay. The message has been imprinted on your mind and will be with you when you continue on your way. In the middle of the many paths with all their confusing events, here is this one path on which you pursue your journey steadfastly.[14]

At the castle people are waiting for the sun, for the circle with the many paths has always been under the sign of the sun.[15] Could it be that the time has come for the sun to break through? For a little while longer the waiting must continue: it is still too cold outside. When the time is ripe, the people will be able to return to their village and they will know why all these things had to be.

Meanwhile you understand the hint: the branch can be planted now, on top of the roof, as house builders do when they have reached the ridge of the roof. Clearly, the time has come.

The Three-Leaf Clover

All around me there are fields and ditches. It is warm, and wherever I look I see clover leaves. They are big, each with three round leaves. There is much to be seen in those leaves. The veins give an impression of roads. I feel as though I am getting smaller and land on one of those clover leaves.

Then the image changes and I am in a hilly landscape with undulating green. There are many trees. The sky is an even blue. It is fine, bright weather but there is no sun to be seen.

I walk through the hills. There are houses with roofs of grass that are barely noticeable. They look just like the hills. It is only when I am right in front of them that I can see they are houses with people inside them, round people. Beside one of the houses there are some big children. In front of the house, on a seat, are a father and a mother. They talk differently from the way I do, but they look friendly. When I come closer they carry on talking without seeing me.

I am closer to the parents than to the children and I go up to them even closer. Then, suddenly, when I cross a certain boundary, they see me. They are waiting for me to approach. The mother holds out her hand. Too many eyes are fixed on me, looking at me. I can't go any farther. Now I ask the children to go away. They do so. Only the parents are still left.

I come closer.

The light disappears. I am still held back.

When the light has gone, she touches me. Then she waits again. I can't raise my hand. The mother is warm.

I want to touch her now. It grows dark and then I take her hand. I have given her my hand and she takes hold of it with both her hands. I hear her voice. Everything is all right.

When I am stuck again she moved up a little, to make more room. Then I take his hand as well.

Now I let them go again but I remain at the same distance. Beside the house a table has been set. On it there are things to eat. They have been expecting me. I cry.

Then I am sitting under a big tree. It has the eyes of the Eternal One. All the sounds are very soft. He smiles.

A Boundary Crossed

So there it is, you have taken a decisive step. It seems that this is what all the waiting was for: the conquest of your fear. All those times when we hoped that your fear would leave you, it did not happen. Again and again those terrible things assailed you, but they have made you stronger within.

Now the time has come. The three-leaf clover was the introductory image. What could it mean? Very soon it became clear: a daughter has returned. One and two make three. The separation had occurred because of fear, the return became possible when the phantom was banished. The talisman was not a simple remedy. The people were ready to receive you. The question was whether you wanted to meet them. Look at them standing there, by their little houses tucked away amid the green. If you didn't want to see them you had every opportunity to avoid them. But you came too close to them and what you could not know is that here everything is determined by distances. The words that were spoken acquired their meaning by virtue of the distance. Far away was cold and nearby was warm and friendly.

When you crossed the first boundary they caught sight of you. A few more steps and they stretched out their hands toward you. Further than that they did not go. It was up to you whether you wanted to take their hands or not. All the last impediments were removed: the younger people disappeared from sight and the light was dimmed. And then it happened: you took the decisive step and grabbed their hands.

It was a strange experience, especially when the table was laid for three. You belonged there. Two people made it clear to you that they loved you. But stranger still was the fact that you understood the message. Very briefly you could let the knowledge enter your mind that their feelings for you were truly meant, and you were able to accept this.

If you didn't know it yet, the images make it abundantly clear that you are on the right track. A table for three, that is a sign not to be misunderstood. Moreover, soon you were sitting under a big tree and hidden among the branches there were the eyes of the Eternal One. His smile accompanies this whole sequence of events.

You are wise enough to realize that one swallow does not make a summer, but it does make a spring. Time to go in search of the shed with the seeds. With an easy mind we can conclude the story here, knowing that all the roads will lead to a circle. The map shows that there will be several more side tracks. I think you are lucky that these will all lead to the one road.

3 – ANSWERS TO THE CHALLENGES OF A CIVILIZATION

In the Wood

A wood full of sturdy trees.
A red hat with white pompoms.
The wolf slinks among the trees.
I walk between the two.
Then a parachute with a toy bear comes down from the sky.
The three of us picnic on the grass.
Little Red Ridinghood and the wolf have a romp. She is a
    match for him.
He lies on his back resting, his legs in the air.

The sun goes down.
I hear the cows lowing.
I think of fishes.

An airplane comes diving down.
The pilot hands a white lace dress to the wolf.
The plane comes down by parachute, as a toy for Little Red
    Ridinghood.

Along the edge of the wood walks an old woman with a
    faggot.
The moon is shining.
The woman eats of the leftovers and licks her fingers.
A swan flies overhead.

When we say goodbye the woman gives me a gold coin.
On it is a picture of a naked dancing girl in peacock feathers.

A rabbit shows me the way to the wild boars' den.
A hero is fighting the leader there.
The hogs are sleeping like bananas.
On the back of one of them I start on a journey.
In the square I see a wedding drenched in the rain.
Frog's eyes stare at me from a puddle.
The deer sprints past at full speed.
At the farm the harvest is piled up.
The farmer and his wife look as if to say: this is not in your
    line.
I stroke the horse which is looking me in the eye.
We understand each other.

THE GREAT CONFUSION

You were in search of yourself. But in the tangle of contradictions
no clear pattern could be detected or construed. As a result you
were also unable to find a more or less satisfactory way of living.
Discussions went on until deep in the night, to try and combine
all the irreconcilable parts into one whole. The confusion grew
ever greater.

In this therapy, you said, one thing must on no account be
allowed to happen: to start talking and analyzing and theorizing
all over again. At the beginning of the therapy you were unable
to present a reasonably complete picture of your problems. You
had more than enough of trying to do that. This led you to direct
your eye inward for a change, and to make contact with your
inner imaginal world. As the story in the wood shows, that world
is at least as chaotic as you believe it to be. But it has one advantage: time and again we are asked to act in this inner world, not
just to think. Thinking is a good thing, but right after the thinking, something has to be done.

When you began with the imaginations, you were thirty-six years old. You are a man who likes adventures. But had you ever expected this adventure? Your choice would probably have fallen on something different, but never mind, it doesn't look as if you are having much trouble with it. Clearly you are not being watched here by any human eyes that might deter you from doing what occurs to you: you walk between the wolf and Little Red Ridinghood. You notice that from time to time there are moments when you are not exactly sure what you should do. If you wait too long, a different image appears and this causes confusion. Yet all the images have something to do with you, even though it is not always immediately clear what they signify. Whoever is going to read them will have difficulties with them. Perhaps we should therefore explain how we have proceeded. At first we understood only a few things. We did not need to know any more at that stage in order to move ahead.

Here and there an image stands out, for instance, the one of the pigs, because you had a horrible, sadistic dream about it. It meant something to you and it was a good thing to settle accounts with the leader of the pigs. Then there was the horse, which deigned to look at you in your loneliness, a look that became one of mutual understanding. You said nothing to each other, and yet there was, from within, an experience of understanding and trust.

The main anchorage in the chaos was that which you yourself began to undertake in the world of images. You felt intuitively that it was necessary to walk between the wolf and Little Red Ridinghood. The wolf's white dress made you even more wary than you already were: he might pretend to be nicer than he really was. And you joined battle with the pig.

As far as the other characters are concerned, we assumed that they would appear in the sequel to the story, and this did indeed happen. Beside the confusion in your thinking, there was also that other confusion in real life, after the encounter with a young woman had stirred up all kinds of thoughts in you with which you didn't know how to cope. You clung to her desperately. When she nevertheless went her own way, you were upset. Such an incident is enought to make you start sharpening the knives, but it also caused everything around you to become misty and seem useless. What was the point of trying to achieve anything in this world? Of course, you have possibilities of achieving something, but it must serve some purpose as well. In this period you no longer saw this so sharply. There was no longer any firm ground under your feet. Every choice took on an air of randomness. What will you decide to do for a living, if you don't even know who you are? You could choose so many professions: journalist, development worker, lecturer. The time to make a choice has not yet come. You had better work on a farm for a while, as you are doing at the moment. Because it does you good to feel earth between your fingers. At this moment everything else will have to be pushed aside. It can wait, although the "musts" are pursuing you. All your life so far has been one long sequence of "musts": always rushing from one thing to the next to show that you could hold your own in the rat race, always focusing on the outside world. Finding all kinds of things important, and then finally discovering that you have become alienated from yourself and that a feeling of total emptiness has come over you. Your brain racks itself trying to gather up all the loose ends as best it can. But it is a hopeless task. Everything is in contradiction to everything else. The confusion is total.

This then is our starting point: many possibilities, little anchorage. It is the starting point for a long journey through yourself. You will get to know the geography of a more than earthly existence, and you will also travel in cosmic spaces. The journey will be exclusively yours, and yet on the other hand it won't. Especially at the beginning, there are many images and experiences that you share with people from previous generations and with present-day people from other parts of the world: the sun sets and the moon rises. We can therefore use the wisdom of all ages. The goddess is bound to make herself known and in her you will meet yourself. The swan that is near her has already shown itself. And you have been given a teddybear to take to bed with you, and not for nothing. Finally there is a gold coin, which predicts something good, even though we are not allowed to know what. It is time to dive under water and we shall see where we surface next.

Behind the Keyhole

I see a long tunnel under water through which I am being sucked at great speed. It frightens me, I see large fishes in the water, and something else. It is a Greek vase with two handles. Two people are depicted on it, in a bright purple color. There is also a date on it, but I can't read what it says. The vase is closed off tightly with a cork. There must be a magic potion in it. I can take it up to the surface with me, but for some reason or other it belongs here, down below. With the aid of a hypodermic needle I try to taste some of the liquid. The world becomes lighter. As through an invisible wall of a dome a different world becomes visible.

There is a keyhole built into a window pane. Through it I see a woman dressed in white, who is busy making a cake. There are several people there, including a man and two children and then this woman in white, in a hoop skirt and a blue blouse. She looks like a chatelaine. There are chandeliers along the wall and there is a great deal of laughter. To judge by the noise there are many more people. The interior is sober, almost Spartan, as in a medieval castle.

When I enter I see the same kind of vase standing there as earlier on under the water. From time to time a little of the contents of the vase is mixed into the food. In the kitchen is a stairway leading to the cellar. There is not much light down there, and smutty things are going on. It is dusty, and there are people having sex together. It is a storage cellar. You are supposed to go around naked there. I hear smacking noises and people are being sucked off. They are things of the flesh there, with a lost of slime and slurping. There is also a door into the slaughter room.

The chatelaine comes down the stairs and shakes hands with

me, she is very friendly but at the same time self-possessed and resolute. "Nice of you to have come," she says, "we were expecting you." I have to go back to the room upstairs. She has her own program and what happens next is this: she points to a kind of desk at which I have to sit down. There are pens lying on it and paper, but when you open a lid a keyboard appears, as of a piano. Now she is standing beside me in the sea green light, her hands folded on her stomach, level with a band of sunlight. She looks expectant. It is very clear what she expects of me. I have to find out what my task is here. It might be to make music or to write texts or both.

Meanwhile my thoughts are with a pretty girl with bare breasts who is lying in a bed. The bed is in the same room. She is calling something like "Come on, then." Clearly they take these things quite casually here. I needn't bother about the stuff on the desk for a while. The chatelaine, however, expects something of me. Are those two each other's opposite poles? Is an and-and possible? I have to sit and think about that. What does she want of me now?

The girl in the bed is a quiet and mild-mannered creature. She has an air of earthiness about her and as far as I am concerned I don't mind if she doesn't say anything. I see through her essence. We make love without immediately heading for the full works. And yet in a very natural way I am now inside her, except it is more a question of our whole bodies rather than just our genitals. It gives me a good feeling. This is something I have been longing for. It has to do with tenderness. The chatelaine has seen it all and she has not shown any disapproval. This fits in with her whole attitude. But the way she stands there indicates that she is expecting more of me than this. She sees it more as a template for what she wants from me next. She points to the desk so I take a seat again, although I still don't know what I am supposed to do there. When I tell her this she replies, "Well, it's lying in front of you, isn't it?" I look all over the desk but I see nothing but pen nibs and the like. She herself sets to work. She has thrown me back on myself. I have a good mind to get back into the bed with the girl, and I do. The chatelaine casts a glance in our direction, which seems to mean something like: just as I thought! So I go back to the desk and jot down a few notes.

The house obviously has another floor. From there you have a good view. A man sits there, busy observing all kinds of things. Somehow or other there are secret systems in this house that serve to maintain communications between the various floors. On the first floor there are holes in the floorboards through which you can look down into the cellar, and for the rest there is something like a pneumatic mail tube alongside the wall. This man (upstairs) never goes downstairs. He presses buttons and then somebody knows he has to go upstairs. I myself belong mainly on the first floor. This is the dullest part. The man upstairs is sitting in a swivel chair. He does not look at me. His attention is totally aimed at the outside. He determines facts and says it is quiet today. What strikes me is that he has been looking in only one direction all the time. Now I notice that just for one instant he is surprised, for he had obviously not seen anything approaching. There are all kinds of obstacles up here, which prevent him from looking in another direction. He is about to start tidying a few things away, but he does not have enough peace and quiet, just like me, when I have to carry out tasks. I can understand his problem and feel a sense of solidarity with him. Mere hard work will not help him. Together we manage to turn a cupboard on its side. The view already becomes a little more open as a result. Tidying away some of the junk will perhaps help as well. Now we really have a better view. The man is satisfied. We have tidied up the side where the moon rises and therefore also the sun. But the man is still an awful dry stick, sitting here all by himself observing. The chatelaine lives very differently. She is the only one who visits all the floors.

When I come outside I see a mailman approaching with a letter for the chatelaine. She opens the letter and reads it. She bursts out in sobs and runs back indoors. Screaming she rushes about the house. Everybody is being stirred up and egged on, for which purpose she uses the letter as a rod. It is quite obvious that she is not ashamed of showing her emotions. It is all hands on deck now. When I ask the girl what is going on she replies she doesn't really know either, but that the whole basis for the existence of the house seems to be in danger.

While I am reflecting on this, I come to the conclusion that something fundamental has to change in the house. They have all started tidying up now, just as we did on the upper floor previously. The old junk is thrown out in a heap. They paint the whole place white, with a hint of blue in it to ward off the flies. The basement area is also dealt with. It is being completely rearranged. There is now a table in it, with one candle standing on it.

But the danger has not yet altogether gone. A black knight approaches, who is going to take charge. It seems high time for me to leave the house. From a distance I hear him giving orders. Suddenly I am seized by a suspicion that he too has crept into bed with the girl. The very thought makes me furious, and I rush into the house to catch the knight. He fights back and tries to impress me with words, but I take no notice of that. Then I see him toppling into a deep pit and the whole house heaves a sigh of relief. It is clear that everyone saw him as a danger. They say that he knew my weak spot but was greatly mistaken.

I myself feel that I should now go to the girl. I want to know where I stand with her. She is still in the bed, half raised, her eyes cast down. Clearly she is embarrassed about the whole affair and says that the knight aroused in her a very great passion, and she adds that I am not able to offer her this. I am too spiritual.

I slink away, disappointed, and start helping the chatelaine washing the dishes. But then my anger at her betrayal rises again and I decide to throw her out of the house. Working with the chatelaine has given me a little more self-confidence.

The House of the Soul

So that is how it happened: a small sip of a magic potion down
there on the bottom of the sea, and the result is that the whole
house of your soul stands in front of you.[1] Your first reactions
suggest that you are largely unfamiliar with the house. It seems
to you as if you are visiting other people. At the beginning it
looked as if you only wanted to look through the keyhole. However, you have to find out that looking means becoming involved
in the drama that takes place behind the door. It must have been
a strange sensation to enter the house, as if you were on an excursion in a medieval building and somebody pulled at your sleeve
and told you that you were expected. The chatelaine came to
meet you just in time, for you were on dangerous terrain. It is
possible to cast a glance into the basement but who among us is
trained to do that these days? We have gotten into the habit of
banishing or denying the instinctive forces of nature and you can
see for yourself what kind of situation that leads to. Slaughter is
taking place down there and you become nauseated when you see
the nadir of sexual experience.

Up the stairs therefore, to the ground floor. Strange things are
happening there as well, but the chatelaine thinks it best to start
work at that place. Soon there are a few things that strike you:
the same drink as there was on the bottom of the sea is here being
mixed with the food, and although you have mentioned that there
is a man in the house, everything seems to be dominated by the
lady of the house. In a very natural way she takes charge of the
events you witness. It is as though we have returned to ancient
times, when in society and in life in general the female element
was much more in the foreground than now. In those days this
woman would probably have been called the primeval mother or
the mother goddess.[2]

Let us see therefore what plans she has for you. It must be said
that she handles the situation in a resolute way. It seems that with
a minimum of instructions you have to find out how you are supposed to arrange your life. In this way she is aiming at a central

problem in your life: what is the purpose of your existence and what will be your contribution to society? You have been unable to find a direction in your life. Although you have studied all kinds of subjects, so many contradictions have been awakened in you that so far you have not succeeded in experiencing all these things as a united whole. You lack a central focus from which everything can be organized. Now it seems that all things are aimed at such a central point.

In the sea green light and with her hands in front of a band of sunlight: that is how she stands before you. She is clearly the mistress of the sea of the unconscious and radiates warmth, energy, and power. She is very direct, you say; you have to find out what your task is. Just as in real life you have numerous possibilities before you, so you now sit at this piano-desk.

In such situations the temptations are great. Is this imaginal situation not very true to nature? Now that you have encountered in one woman a totally new world, the lid is off. All your feelings and urges have broken loose in you at once and you have lost control over them. On the other hand, many good things have got under way at the same time. By her tender touch, the woman was able to take you to your feelings. Unfortunately for you, she then left you again, in the midst of the confusion.

How easily you then move back to the embrace of the young woman in the four-poster bed. As usual, it is the way in which others look at you that has to show you decisively whether or not you are doing the right thing. The chatelaine does not look at you with disapproval and this is the sign that you are doing all right. The second time, however, she looks at you a little more critically. Your progress at the piano-desk is not particularly good, although you have made some discoveries there, because you very often wonder about two aspects that are important to you: rhythmical sounds have done you a lot of good of late, they have brought you closer to yourself, while on the other hand it is a great wish of yours to be able to express yourself clearly in language. For the time being, then, there is a deadlock. Time to continue the journey through the house. On the upper floor you encounter the most recognizable part of yourself. The intellectual, who registers facts with a critical eye and is startled out of his mind when something unexpected occurs. However, we are concerned here not only with the intellectual and his shortcomings, but also with the tendency of many people to hold man's intellectual, analytical powers in such high esteem that the other side of life is lost from sight. In the language of the old myths this is expressed as follows: everything is dominated by the sun and by the male element; compared with this the moon and the female element are pushed into the background.

In addition, you make yet another discovery: the man never goes downstairs, he lives altogether in his head and knows only by hearsay that he also has a body. Very ingeniously an external communication system has been devised, by means of a pneumatic mail system, whereby you remain up to date with what your body has to tell you, but without having any direct contact with it. Music must indeed be of great benefit to you. Music takes you straight back to your links with the earth.

So much for your examination of the situation in which you find yourself. Most of the points of recognition you found in the man upstairs. He lacks the peace and quiet to put order into his affairs and to clear away the obstacles that obstruct his view of the other half of life, that of the nocturnal sky. It is at this point that you intervene. Putting the cupboard in a horizontal position clears the view of the moon. In a symbolic way you thereby bring the influence of the moon and the moon goddess into the house, who, in the far distant past, occupied such a central position in civilizations several thousands of years BC.[3] At the same time, however, this would mean that the influence of the chatelaine, who is closely related to the moon goddess, is extended to the upper floor. The question arises whether this can indeed be done, or whether it is not an all too radical intervention. After all, those ancient civilizations were followed by thousands of years in which the male element was central, and was placed in the foreground, if need be with violence, in the name of the true faith. This intervention would imply the introduction of a totally different attitude toward life in you. An attitude whereby not so much intelligence or the I.Q. is the measure of all things, but the E.Q., the Eros Quotient.[4] This is the capacity for loving, although we have not yet devised a figure to indicate how clever we are at that. It is in particular the influence of the moon goddess that used to bring people closer to themselves and to each other and allowed them to be aware of their connection with the cosmos.

If all this is about to happen in you, you have your work cut out, and if I were you I would go downstairs, for it is not impossible that resistance is already being organized down there. Vested interests do not so easily allow themselves to be dislodged.

You saw it happen. The whole house was in a state of turmoil, when the black knight within you had risen in order to turn the tide. The chatelaine is all to pieces and has hastily ordered the basement to be swept and whitewashed. The paint is white, with a tinge of blue, to ward off the flies, you say. Once again the flies are to be blamed. Even in biblical times the lord of the flies, called Beelzebub, was put to the fire and the sword.[5] The goddesses were taken to the dung heap and women were demoted to second-class citizens.

The recent developments that had taken place in you came within a hair's breadth of being reversed. The knight seized control and unleashed a profound passion in the woman in the four-poster bed. And in doing so he went just that little bit too far. You were on the point of leaving the field, but now you intervened in order to rescue whatever could be salvaged. You will have to start afresh, but it seems that you have made your choice.

A New Phase for the People

I am sitting on the roof of a church. A slater is at work there, because the rain was coming into the church. We are on an island here. In the distance I can see another tower, which looks somewhat like Big Ben. Not another church, I hope? A bell is ringing. You can hear it across the sea. Suddenly we are in a

hurry. The slater and I hasten to get down, to the boat. There
is also a woman there, and the three of us quickly jump into
the boat.

On the open sea I see sharks swimming underneath the boat.
Meanwhile my attention has been distracted. Where were we
going again? Oh yes, that bell. I now see that many small boats
are sailing in the same direction. Fortunately, the slater is a calm
sort of man. He is simply present. Like the spokes of a wheel
the boats converge on the island where the bell tower is. The
ringing sounds unpleasantly loud now. It is indeed a church. I
don't like that, for I detest everything to do with churches and
with Catholicism. The church stands on top of a rock. We have
to climb a number of steps.

At the top of the hill is a plateau. Lots of sheets have been
spread out on the grass there. People are sitting around them.
Music begins to play softly. The scene is not only cheerful but
also important. A Russian Orthodox priest has something to say.
He seems an unpleasant fellow. I shudder at the sight of him.

What is happening here has something to do with a new
phase in the lives of the people. A new step has to be taken.
This requires watchfulness and effort. From the church tower,
lines are sent down with decorations on them. Where exactly
they have to go is not clear to me. Of course, I could ask the
priest about it, but I prefer to talk to someone from the
orchestra. He says it has something to do with the moon. It is
not merely a question of distance or anything like that. It is
going to be an entirely new chapter. Something like: the moon
is going to describe a different orbit around the earth. And the
influence of the moon will also be more directly and more
consciously noticeable. All the people are sitting in the dark
around the sheets, waiting for the moon. It rises late. It must be
a full moon. The moon brushes past the top of the tower and is
now exactly behind the cross. This is annoying, but true. The
people are singing and hold one another by the hand. We three
do the same. The moon now descends slowly. And wanes. Only
now do I see what has happened. It had risen as a waxing moon,

became full behind the cross, and is not setting as a waning moon. The whole cycle completed in one night. It sinks with its convex side touching the horizon first. The earth trembles briefly and then it is time to go back.

For Whom the Bell Tolls

The roof of the church leaks, of course that is no news to you. In some way or other a tremendous resistance has risen in you, against the traditional collective faiths, but as a result you are now wandering around as one who is spiritually homeless. And yet it won't leave you in peace, you want to find your own meanings. At the beginning of this imagination we therefore find you in the company of the slater on the roof of the church, but he does not have any answers either. Albeit with reluctance, the two of you set off on the road when in the distance a bell is rung. From the way so many little boats are heading for the same place, you conclude that something drastic is about to happen, even though you have no idea what it might be.

When you arrive by the second church, it begins to dawn on you: a new phase is about to start for the people. This is a strange remark, because you don't say that a new phase is beginning for you, but for the people. It can't therefore be a question of a new kind of faith, because that would normally concern only a small part of mankind. On inquiry it turns out that the moon needs to be closely watched, because its influence on mankind is about to increase significantly. Although you have found a good vantage point for this purpose, it takes some while before it dawns on you how exactly this change is being represented in images. The cross had distracted your attention, but at last you get the message: all the phases of the moon become visible in one single night.[6]

In the previous story you had already taken steps to clear the view of the moon, but at that time you did not yet know that such a radical, symbolic event was to take place. Perhaps it was a good thing that your attention was fixed on the cross for so long, because at least that means it has not escaped you that for a brief moment the cross and the full moon coincided and became one symbol. In the past this was usually a sign that the equilibrium between the different forces in the universe, such as the forces of the four elements: water, fire, air, and earth, and also male and female, was in jeopardy.[7] It might therefore be useful to pay closer attention to this in the future.

An increase in the influence of the moon can, of course, already be observed to some extent, in such things as the women's movement and the increasing concern for the fate of the environment and the survival of human life in general.

Here in your case we may expect that the influence of the female pole both in the conscious and the unconscious part of your Self will increase considerably.

The Scorpion

The term *moon dance* comes to my mind. I would prefer not to think of dancing. The name was a good one, though. I see that someone is dancing, but it is not one of the people who are here with me. It is a woman in rags, as in an Indian temple. I see her dancing in the fire, and there are flashes of lightning in the sky. She beckons me to join in, but I immediately suppress that fanciful idea. Yet it will not leave me alone. There is a point of conflict in me. If only I could do it safely, but that fire seems very hot to me. I know I am going to do it all the same. If only there was some music for me to hide behind.

There is no stopping me, I am already dancing. Everybody starts to clap rhythmically and there are drums and congas. She dances in the Indian fashion while I dance more like an African, wilder therefore. But it is okay. The people are forming a circle that comes closer and closer. Normally I would be afraid to be so surrounded. Here it is all right. It is very special, to be dancing like this in a fire. The people are making a trellis of their spears above our heads. Suddenly the woman has vanished. I grab hold of the spears and am carried to a river.

There they lower me. It hisses. So far everything has gone well. The trellis is laid on the river, so that it becomes a raft on which I sail away in the direction of the sea.

In the sea there is a rock sticking out above the water. That is where I have to go and also the people who are with me on the raft. On the island there is a palm tree. Near it someone sits tailor-style. It is a woman. She has a sturdy body. She says, "Hi, so you have arrived." She is there because of us. She is not a slut. She is someone with self-respect. She possesses a certain kind of freedom. When we have become used to the surroundings we see that the woman is carrying out a certain ceremony. She is sharing out something. It has to do with fire, because she is preparing something in a cooking pot. It bubbles and has to do with a scorpion. The scorpion is in a little cage, close by. We all have to take a sip from the potion.

I think she must be a sorceress or a priestess. She gets up and comes toward me. Then she places the scorpion on my head. It crawls down over my nose, buries itself inside my shirt and walks down, right across my prick, and stings me in the balls. It doesn't hurt very much. In a sense it makes you potent. Then the scorpion crawls upward across my back. When all this is finished the woman beckons me and I have to do it with her. I feel as if I were busy with a she-bear. I don't know why this is, because she is really a woman. But she has the same kind of firmness about her.

THE INITIATION INTO THE UNCONSCIOUS

Your study of the house of the soul has brough to light several important things. In the first place a very one-sided intellectual activity was being carried out on the upper floor, without having any counterpart in the form of intuition which knows without being able to indicate how the knowledge is acquired. Secondly, in the basement the instincts had free rein and there was nobody to keep matters under control. You know this part of yourself and it worries you. Sometimes everything comes together in a single experience, for example when you walk past the butcher's store in the village of your birth and old childhood memories come to mind. You were seized by panic when you could hear the screaming of the pigs being slaughtered, while at the same time it made you so excited that you had an erection as a result. You were totally incapable of controlling the forces that raged in you at such times.

In addition you are at this moment especially aware of the outbursts of aggression that enable you to wipe the floor with everyone and everything and make a clean sweep. The black knight is also a familiar figure to you. Injustice always tends to make you very angry and you are sorely tempted to do away with democracy for a while and issue the necessary orders from above.

Against this background it is worth having a closer look at all the things that happen in the story of the scorpion. Unfortunately our knowledge of the ancient symbolic imagery in this story is still very inadequate. We shall have to make do with the small bits that are at our disposal.

To start with, there is the moon dance, which did indeed occur in the rituals connected with the moon goddess, although in a rather different way from your experience here.[8] What fascinated people most about the moon was the phenomenon of its changing shape, its waxing and waning, whereby the most frightening moment was the time when the moon could not be seen at all. In the moon dance this waxing and waning of the moonlight was embodied, and it was in this way people, by means of a dance, came to terms with the great mystery surrounding these changes. The most striking aspect of your moon dance is the woman who dances in the fire. You draw a connection between her and an Indian temple. This is a second indication that we are here dealing with a very special dance. It is a ritual dance, by means of which a psychological event is being enacted. In India, the dancing god Shiva was indeed surrounded by a circle of flames, to indicate that an incarnation of eternal energy was taking place. So there again there was proof that people can truly become part of a much larger happening. Heaven and earth may be separated, but they can be experienced as parts of one united whole. And the same is true of the reality that men and women are separate but can experience each other as united together.

You have had to conquer many things before you were able to take part in this fire-dance ritual. The fire is frightening and in the world outside it is only possible in very exceptional circumstances to be in a fire and not burn yourself. In this imaginal world, however, it is possible, and you must have suspected something of this, otherwise you would not have ventured into the fire. And then there are a few more small details: you are not a very good dancer, and then to dance with so many people around you is not at all an easy thing to do. Yet you are pulled into it. "I know I am going to do it," you say, and that is how it is. Then the events follow one another in quick succession. The people make a kind of trellis or net on which you are lowered into the river. In this way aggression is put aside and two images are combined which in the ancient feminine civilization used to occur in so many images: the net and the water, as a sign that we are dealing with living water or, if you like, life-giving water. According to this train of thought, life originated from water. So you sail toward the open sea in your remarkable conveyance. You have learned a great deal about how to give events a chance, and you have even become very curious to find out what all this is leading to. You want to know. Together with a few friends you are furthermore prepared to deal with the strange world of the unconscious. "Hi, so you have arrived," someone says. It was not a coincidence then, the events fit in with a specific plan. To start with, you are given something to drink and you have some idea of how this drink was made.

If this tree is the moon tree, as can be seen in pictures from the ancient past, and if this woman is the priestess who mediates in the encounter with the moon goddess, then the potion can also be identified. It would have to be the soma potion, which people used to be given to drink in this ceremony, made of sea water and the fruit of the moon tree.[9] This soma was the source of inspiration for the development of the Self, as an inner voice that pos-

sessed a natural wisdom. If all this is true, then it could be the
introduction to an inner movement toward controlling the un-
bridled instinctive forces in the basement of the house.

Many men have seen her before, this lonely woman, usually
high up in the mountains, and many have wondered whether this
is a suitable sort of place for a woman on her own. In your case
she is on a solitary rock. You seem to take it for granted that she is
there, but you are surprised at the strange fashion of her dress
and at the scorpion in a cage which she has with her.

Perhaps here we should say a little more about that lonely
woman in the mountains or, as others call her, "the lady of the
animals."[10]

In ancient Greece there is a well-known story of the goddess
Artemis, the goddess of the hunt. She assembled the animals
around her. Unlike the men, she did not fight the animals but
subjected them to her. It was she who gathered young girls and
brought them together in groups in order to initiate them to life,
by involving them in ritual dances. She was clad in bearskins and
the young girls were called the she-bears.[11] She was there also
for the men, although the men could not be her partners. She was
the virgin, the woman who did not belong to men, let alone to
one single man. She was there as the person who knew by nature how to deal with the instinctive forces in mankind, which
were represented by animals. Hence "the lady of the animals."
She knew all about the animal forces in us and knew how to deal
with them.

In view of the circumstances in the basement of the house, it is
not insignificant that you should meet her here. She will probably be able to unleash the counterforce in you which will allow
you to deal with the situation. Clearly, this requires quite an
operation. The sacred animal from Egypt, the scorpion, has to be
brought in to arrange one thing and another. In Egypt there was
a goddess who used to be represented with a scorpion on her
head, and this honor now falls to you.[12] The scorpion itself would
be portrayed with the head of the goddess Isis. So you are in very
distinguished company.

You make no objections. The scorpion's journey over your body would make many other people shudder, but you remain fairly calm under it. It is as though the priestess has made so great an impression on you that you dare to be confident that all will turn out well. Even the potency-enhancing sting you take in your stride. What kind of potency is this, anyway? It can not be ordinary sexual potency, because you tend to have too much of that rather than too little. We must therefore look in the direction of your potency or power to relate to the female power, which presents itself here and which will enable you to cope with the animal element in you, without being devoured by it.

The Women's Archipelago

A dragon ship comes sailing along, with a swan in its sail. My attention is drawn by this swan because it is moving. The swan asks what I am doing on this ship. Indeed I am now on board. I tell him I am on my way to something unknown. It is a voyage of exploration. "Well," says the swan, "then you have done right to choose this ship." I ask why he is hanging in the sail like a crucified Christ. He says, "By being a symbol like this I can have more influence on the course of events." There is something erotic about the swan and also something pure. It has to do with fate and with surrender. The swan has a cut in his neck from which blood is flowing. This has to do with sadness and with destiny.

I grab hold of an oar in order to lend destiny a hand. I am in a hurry to make sure that events take their proper course. When I look back from the forward deck I see the world gliding away from us. We are sailing into space. The ship moves forward like the swan itself, with stretching movements of the dragon's head. The ship sails rhythmically. The rhythm seems to be important. We sail in the opposite direction of the setting sun. Tall grass rises out of the water. There is something like an island, where only women live. Their special quality is that they can walk on

the water. It is a kind of women's commune. They have their
own social organization. They live from what the sea supplies.
There are several more islands, all belonging together.

They don't mind us going ashore. We go to their island in
order to learn something about how they conduct their lives.
There is something special, something mysterious about them,
apart from the fact that they can walk on water. I have an idea
that they have something to do with festivals and with the
supernatural. But I can't find out about that just yet. They rule
the whole area. There is also a queen. We are given a hospitable
reception. They knew we were coming. What a pity that I am
unable to discover their secret.

In some way or other these island women have a secret, and
this secret forms the core of their special life. It is a kind of
power, but how or what exactly is unclear to me.

The men with whom I am in the boat split up so that each
woman has a guest. I am visiting a woman of a somewhat
Oriental appearance. She radiates a certain sensuality. She seems
to do everything in a crouched position. She has coal black eyes
and a rare combination of thinness and yet soft rounded curves.
Mmmm, a delicious hostess.

In the course of the evening it appears that she, like me, has a
desire to make love. Before we go to bed, something most
extraordinary happens: she crouches down with her feet flat on
the ground, as those Oriental women can do so casually . . . and
takes a mussel out of her cunt. Then she comes to me. I am
utterly astonished. This must have something to do with their
secret and with the central point of their organization. It seems
that when they make love they briefly put aside their special
powers and become ordinary beings of flesh and blood. At any
time they can resume their special powers. I find this a difficult
idea to get used to and I dare not do as I please. This way,
making love acquires an air of being used.

The following morning I decide to have a talk with her about
one thing and another. She says she is not allowed to reveal the
secret, but that it is accessible to anyone who discovers it for

himself. Nothing is kept hidden. The mussel has something to do with it, but it works only, for instance as a contraceptive, when you know the secret. She also discloses that they worship a godhead or a power that resides under water. But for the rest I have to discover it all by myself. They keep nothing concealed. The secret is accessible to anyone who is receptive toward it and is ripe for it. They themselves also had to discover it on their own, but because they chose to live in this commune for a time, they underwent a period of training which has sharpened their powers of observation of certain aspects of life. She admits that this is more difficult for men.

The next morning my mates from the dragon ship leave the island. I have decided to stay here, because I want to know more about it. Time and time again I want to discover truths about life. I have often gotten into trouble and various crises as a result. But here it seems to be different. Here it seems more of an adventure. In the past the meaning of my life seemed to depend on it. That is still so now, but you could say that this time I can only win. If I don't discover the secret I am no worse off than when I first arrived here. I want to share in the secret of the women and I am also prepared to offer a service in return, as long as I can stay here on these islands.

When the men leave, the captain calls out: "Think of your own boat! Discovering secrets is fun, but being your own boss is worth something too." The swan in the sail winks at me. A feeling of nostalgia takes possession of me and also a feeling of loneliness, being all on my own surrounded by nothing but women. But never mind, it also has an attractive side.

Now I am walking on the main island and I arrive behind the hut of the queen, in the central square. There I catch a few words ". . . and then you must make sure he is wearing the sacrifical clothes and that somehow he arrives here on the main island, then we can overpower him."

In a state of some bewilderment I now wander about on the island of the dark woman. I intend to talk about it with her: what was the meaning of this and what it was all about and who

it was about. A moment later the woman appears, but there is
no opportunity to ask any questions, for she is busy with
something. However, there is every reason to be suspicious, for
what other "he" could there possibly be on these islands except
me? Then the woman takes a garment out of a box and says,
"Here, do me a favor. Put on these pants and wear them for as
long as you are here. I'd like you to do that." I examine the
pants and see to my surprise a hole on either side of the crotch,
as big as an egg. If I were to put on these pants, my two balls
would peep out through these holes. Well, that makes it crystal
clear to me who and what they are intending to sacrifice, and
how. I also realize with a shock what their secret is, roughly:
once a year they sacrifice a fellow who is mad enough to want to
discover their secret, and it looks as if now it is just about the
right moment. So I am the one who has to walk into the trap. I
say to the woman, "Okay, I'll go and change my clothes."
Meanwhile I reflect that it would be rather exciting to walk
about in those pants and make love. I know that there is no
danger as long as I am not on the main island.

So I go back to the woman in my balls-pants. She laughs and
grabs me by the balls. As I thought, making love is great like
this.

But afterward it is high time for me to get away. On a pretext
I make myself scarce, I gently glide into the water and swim
away, out to sea. What next? For some reason or other I am full
of high spirits. I am sure something good will turn up. Actually,
I had expected more of these women, more answers to my
questions and a clearer revelation of their secret. Perhaps this
was not the right place for it.

THE THREATS OF THE UNCONSCIOUS

To go on a voyage through our inner world is an exciting adventure. The inner world is one in which there are many temptations
but also a number of dangers. As regards the latter, there is a difference whether the journey is made as a man or as a woman. You

make the journey as a man, and this means that the unknown world of the unconscious will appear to you chiefly in a female form, as we have seen so far.

Now that the initiation rites are over, the actual voyage can begin. You are on board a dragon ship, together with only men, and this at once indicates a whole program of what may be expected. The mother ship and the mother dragon, full of inexperienced men, not counting the captain and the swan; I am curious to find out what will happen. The swan knows all about it, or so it seems. It is a symbolic swan, you are told, and this means it is a swan with influence. Your fate depends on it. In ancient myth the swan was to be found in the vicinity of Leda, Aphrodite, and Artemis, and so we may assume that the story of your journey will be continued here on this ship.[13]

You are sailing in the direction opposite the setting sun and we may therefore suppose that you are traveling toward the moon. Moreover, it seems as though the ship is leaving the earth. This makes the journey a cosmic one, although the ordinary elements are present, for within a short time there is water once again, and islands are looming up. Women live there separately from men and they have arranged their lives entirely in their own way. It is just the sort of thing you like, to be able to study such an unusual society from close up.

Most of all it is the air of mystery in that place which greatly excites your imagination. What can be the secret of these women? That they are possessed of special powers is immediately obvious to you. Also that you are under the spell of their power? Not quite that, I believe, at least not yet. You more or less feel that you can move in any direction. You still feel free to come and go wherever you please. But if I am not mistaken, it is the freedom of someone who is in love. You think you are still in control, but in fact you are busy burning your boats. Listen to the captain, who is advising you to think of your own boat. The swan winks and so we must assume that nothing will come of it, because the swan controls your fate.

In the reality of every day I hear you complain that sex is dominating your life too much. It is on your mind all the time and you can't stop thinking about it. On these islands it must drive you crazy altogether. Luckily, these things are quite well organized here, so that some kind of order can be created in you as well.

It is as if lovemaking is not simply lovemaking here. The reason for this is that the women are dedicated to their own center, to a power that resides at the bottom of the sea. Besides, they are virgins, that is to say women who have their own lives, and do not exist for the men. At those moments when they wish to meet a man, they put the mussel aside and after making love they pick up their power again and continue to lead their own lives.

Actually, this is a story we could have known before, for did not Aphrodite regularly renew her virginity by immersing herself in the sea, to reappear again carried by the shell of a mussel? [14] Virginity has nothing to do with making love, but with having a center of one's own. Just as men have a center of their own, so women have one too, albeit a different one, as we shall see later. [15]

Your decision has been made, you are staying behind on your own in this archipelago, in search of the secret. Clearly you are not aware of the fact that you might be swallowed up by the mother dragon. Like a spy on foreign soil, you catch a few incoherent statements, which nevertheless arouse a certain disquiet in you. Slowly it dawns on you that a cruel deed is being prepared, but the signs will have to become very clear if you are to give up your plan. You simply can't get enough of the motherly warmth, not even when you are given the ceremonial garment to wear in which the castration is to be carried out.

And yet it is necessary for you to detach yourself from all this nest-warmth.

Luckily for you, you meet several women who are motherly in the favorable sense of the word. They are capable of mustering the necessary hardness to sacrifice their son, so that they themselves are able to live as free women again. And you will be liberated from them to find your own individuality, and after that you will be welcome again. In effect, at a certain moment a woman needs to sacrifice her son by giving up her maternal feelings for him; and a man must put aside his sonship in order to become himself.

Without knowing it, you have begun to appreciate the wisdom of this ancient ritual whereby the goddess annually castrates her son in order that he may live as a free man and choose a wife for himself.[16]

Ouroboros

Swimming in the sea I take off those ridiculous pants. The temptation is too great. The pants sink to the bottom of the sea. A fish darts into them. There is such a wild commotion that for a moment I see nothing. Then I see the fish's head sticking out through one of the holes in the pants. He emerges altogether and then goes back inside through the other hole. It is an eel, and he comes to rest as if riveted like a ring through a nose, peering out through one of the holes.

This was accompanied by tumultuous movement and this is why the great secret beast, which always sleeps in the dark, has woken up. It is a large, reptile-like monster from prehistoric times. He has not quite become a fossil yet, and begins to set himself in motion, rises toward the surface and finds me there: a sprawling naked little human being. He opens his mouth wide and I am swept into it.

Inside him, I arrive in a slimy room. Three men are playing cards by a little table, by the light of a small wick. "Ha, here's another one," they say. "We were just one player short. Have you been with the women too?" "Yes I have," I say, "but how can you people stay alive in here?" "Oh, when you are here, time stands still," they say, "just as it does for the beast himself. The main thing here is that you feed your spirit. You have to get it all out of yourself. But at least you can find peace and quiet here."

Then, out of the darkness of the intestines, clad in animal skins and armed with a club, there appears a Teutonic figure. He is a good-natured guest. He had gone in search of an exit from the labyrinth of the beast, but was unable to find one in all the centuries of his being here. Now the five of us devise a plan to escape. I suggest the idea of making the beast nauseous by dancing around in him. And sure enough, after a while we pass by his molar teeth and float to the surface. The Teuton at once occupies a special position. He has found a mast we can hold onto. The wind carries us in the direction of an island with a tall snow-covered mountain on it. In fact, I don't really want to go to any island just now.

Fortunately, the dragon ship approaches. The captain greets us and it turns out that he knows the Teuton. He says that he and the swan knew all about what happened. He has been cruising in these regions for a long time, but he knows he must not try to stop events from happening. They must run their appointed course. He is glad to see us again.

REBIRTH

In this story you never know whether you are on the way to freedom or whether you are swimming straight into a trap. On the island you were able to escape from a threatening danger but whether you are now back in safe waters is another question. No sooner have you got rid of those peculiar pants than the Ouroboros comes swimming along, the snakelike fish that bites its own tail. In this extraordinary manifestation the snake has become the image of circular time, when has neither beginning nor end. In the world in which that time reigns, you cannot say that death is an end, nor that birth is a beginning. Here dying is a necessary condition for renewal and this is why dying is in fact a form of change.

The world of the soul is governed by this time and the circular snake is therefore the introduction to the impending changes. You will disappear from the surface of the earth and you will return as a different person. The wriggling creature vanishes into the mouth of the huge secret beast, the primordial mother or the dragon, deep down at the bottom of the sea. Thus the devouring power of this mother of creation has caught you in the end.[17] It is difficult to escape from this power when everything is directed toward making sure that you are caught by it. However, all these things do not necessarily mean that the end has come for you. In this place there is no end, everything is eternal. Ordinary time stands still here, but when the correct rituals are performed, everything begins to live once again. A complete waiting room has even been set up and they are short of a fourth person. They all share the same fate and they have therefore known from the start where you have come from. They are unable to tell you much about what is to be done next. There is one thing they know and that is that you must not go in the direction of the labyrinth in the belly of the best. You would never in your life find the way out. Suitable means will have to be found to travel from one reality into the other. Fortunately, you have some experience of this now, and you manage to persuade the others to do a ritual dance inside the monster. This makes the beast feel sick and that is your chance. Like Jonah in the whale you are spewed out, toward the new life.

This means a life in which you stand on your own two feet, not a life in which you are passive, but where you can take your own decisions. It is also a life which adds its own values to the feminine values in which you have just been instructed. This is very necessary if you are to find your way in society.

The Sun Wheel

Smoke is rising from the top of the snow-covered mountain, which is an odd thing to happen to a snow-covered mountain. There are also a lots of little black figures coming out of the top, which then gather together on the beach. There they unfurl a banner, very large and very long. On it is written in big letters: FOR THE RIGHTS OF THE SUN.

Meanwhile I notice that I myself am on the way to the crater, in order to find out what is going on. There is a smithy inside the crater. A tall chimney carries the smoke upward and out. There is a damper in the chimney which makes it possible to send smoke signals. A devilish figure is in charge. His tail ends in the form of a heart. Other figures are poking and stirring the fire with iron pokers. They are making a cartwheel. There is a cart there, which bears some resemblance to a Roman chariot. It is a chariot that carries you through the air. That is what the Teuton and I will do, we will make a voyage through the air in that vehicle. He remains very calm under it. I have to spur on the horses. He hangs over the side of the chariot.

Below us lies the ship. There is a large expanse of sea with an island here and there. We are safe up here, and we debate whether we should fly over the women's island. They can't catch us now anyway. We fly across the island without danger, we are very high above it. The women are lying in the sun. We want to let them know that we have passed overhead. When we are right above them I call out: "The pants are lying in the water."

Now I feel something like a struggle in myself. I want to go down there and at the same time I have a feeling that we have to be very careful indeed. We alight on the water and before long the woman I met on one of the islands comes swimming along toward us. I ask her what exactly was the purpose of those pants. She replies, "We eat up only those who want to be eaten up." Then she explains that we are allowed to mingle with them but that we have to maintain a certain distance. She means that we cannot take part in their lives. "If you are so keen on being completely abosrbed into the world of women, then so you will be." When we take our leave she says, "Always welcome, but now you know the score."

Together, the Teuton and I take the chariot back. We both think the woman is right. And we really needed to know this. It gives us a kind of freedom, while the road to the women has not been cut off. When we are back by the crater we lie down to rest in the four-poster bed. The voyage was well worth the trouble.

On the Road to Adulthood

Your desire to visit yet another island has completely vanished. Yet you are unable to drive the newly occurring image of the island with the white crater into the background. There is probably a meaning behind it, you conclude, and so you decide to go along with this image. With great emphasis it was announced from the beach that "the rights of the sun" were at issue. Clearly this means that you had gone along too far with the influences of the moon. You had a narrow escape from the dangers of your action. Let us therefore have a closer look at what this crater has to offer you.

To begin with, you come upon a classical scene: a large fire and a devil close by it. The fire served to purify people and to liberate them, especially from the influences of this devil.[18] Although you grew up with a belief in the devil and in purgatory, I do not notice that it upsets you in any way. Your interest is immediately directed toward what is being made down there in the fire. You have landed in the world of material things, let us say, the beginning of the world as we know it now. What is important here is that which can be made, the things that can be ready first and those that are made later. People think about causes and effects, they establish rules and they like to have order and regularity. They strive for perfection, and you have to assert yourself with a certain aggressiveness. It is the world of communication and economics.[19]

In normal circumstances, you would not be too keen to enter that world. But your desire for adventure knows no bounds and something very tempting has been set up for you here. A real sun chariot, so that you can whizz through the air in the wake of the god Helios. There are quite a few plans to be forged in this crater. If a wheel can be forged, then obviously many more things are possible. The most desirable objects will shortly be presented to mankind and you will contribute your little mite. But first you will take a trip through the air, and make cautious contact with the women in the archipelago.

The Asian woman is prepared to give some explanation, now

that you have already discovered most of the message yourself. Everything you have experienced on the island, and also in the sequel at the bottom of the sea, formed part of the secret. A second birth was necessary, which was accomplished when you managed to escape from the big fish. It was an age-old rite, which is still today performed on young men in the jungle. To carry out this ceremony, a hut has been built in the shape of a large fish.[20] Afterward you will expand your identity further, but beforehand it was necessary to realize that "being absorbed into the world of women" is not a desirable option for you. The transition to a center of your own is not always pleasant. Sometimes you have to leave a lot behind and the prospects in our men's world are not always very attractive. You will have to find your own way, and the crater offers you a first chance.

In the Cavalry

With boat and all we circle around in a whirlpool and are being sucked down, toward the bottom of the sea. There the boat comes to rest on dry land. We step out of it and can walk across the sand. I poke my finger into the wall of water, and this creates a circle which then becomes horizontal so that we are able to look across the water again.

In the distance we can see a castle which looks like a cream cake. I feel a great sense of doubt rising in me, whether I really want to go there or not. It seems I have wavered for a little too long, for now I see myself already on my way toward it, wading through the water. From one of the towers a white flag has been hoisted with a text written on it which I cannot read. Around the castle a palisade has been erected, such as you often see in Westerns.

Somehow or other I have arrived inside the enclosure, and there I see people busy with horses. They are soldiers. They are wearing round flat caps, each with a cross on the flat part. Again, a cross within a circle.

There is a black horse waiting for me. The other soldiers appear to approve of this. The horse puts his head on my shoulder. This makes me realize how soft the underside of a horse's neck is. I have to take care of this horse now. I am told I have to pay for him, or if I don't I must join this cavalry unit. I am free to come and go as I please. That appeals to me quite a lot, so I decide to join up. I do not have to submit to their discipline, they say. Just as well, I think, because that would not suit me at all.

Like the others, I take up residence in a stable. There is a central kitchen where I can obtain my meals and the next day I have to report for a personal assignment. It seems that I am predestined to carry out certain missions, like, for instance, measuring water levels or things of that kind.

It appears that there are Indians in the neighborhood. They are sending me to these Indians as a messenger, because they seem to think I can probably get on well with them. I must try to develop contact with them. So I set off through a hilly landscape and finally end up in a wood where there is a clearing. A fire is being made in a hold in the ground. Gathered around the fire I see a lot of cripples and lepers. They are in need of vitamins and medicine. I do not want to act out of pity. When I ask them whether they have anything to barter it turns out that they possess no material goods, only peace. It is very peaceful there, and it seems as if these people do not need to achieve anything. My struggle between ambition and doing nothing is stirred by it.

ACTING IN INNOCENCE

Finding yourself in a whirlpool suggests a reorientation. The result is that for the continuation of the drama we find ourselves in the setting of a castle in the form of a frosted cream cake.

And as though this were not enough, there is even an enclosure of palisades, so that the idea of a Western occurs to you. So it turns out to be a mixture of the old-fashioned and contem-

porary romanticism. It appears we are at the beginning of the co-
lonial era. At high speed the entire history of mankind passes before your eyes. Carried along by a spirit of adventure, you forge
ahead and you do not shrink from taking certain risks, as we already noticed earlier in the women's archipelago. Here you join
the cavalry without realizing that by doing so you have come
within reach of all the myths to do with riders and their horses.
You are well on the way to discovering the secrets of this male
society. At once your weakest spot is attacked, your tender feelings for the horse's warm, soft neck. No sooner have these feelings evolved in you than there is talk of payment. And if you are
unable to pay, you may join the cavalry. You spend a brief moment investigating to what extent you are bound by the contract,
and then you probably commit the same error that the whole of
mankind has always made: you become a soldier and you seem to
think that it is possible to be a soldier without being counted as
part of the warring parties.

Your choice is understandable. There is a lot to be said for it.
The state has undertaken to feed you and give you shelter. Furthermore you will probably be given missions to carry out and
this will flatter your vanity. You will be doing harmless tasks,
such as measuring water levels and the like. In doing so you will
be contributing to the "general good," so it is quite all right for
you to take it on.

Meanwhile a profound suspicion has risen in me. Looking at it
from the outside, I have the impression that you are walking into
a trap. It is as though you are going to be used for quite different
purposes from the ones you imagine. The first water levels you
are sent to measure are those of the Indians, and you have soon
drawn your conclusion: the water comes to their lips. They are all
mortally sick. What is to be done? It has become a serious problem: those people have nothing to barter. All they can offer is
tranquillity and relaxation, but what can you buy with that? At
best it is something of use to you personally, and for the rest you
are once again briefly aware of being driven by ambition.

Growing Tomatoes

Now that I am able to observe the state of the forest dwellers from close by, I realize that it cannot go on like this. I travel back and forth to the castle several times and pinch whatever is necessary from the stores in the cellar. An agricultural business is being set up in the woodland area. It appears that the tomato plantation is already producing a surplus.

One morning I am summoned by the commander of the castle. I am being let in through a large gateway. The walls are beautifully decorated with mosaics. Behind a large desk sits the commander, in khaki uniform. I had not expected this in a castle of this sort.

He seems very businesslike, which reassures me. No conflict, therefore. He says, "It has come to my notice that you are in regular contact with the people in the wood. So far we have always kept our distance from them, because we have had difficulties in the past. Our policy is aimed at being nonaggressive, and for the rest we have never been interested in having anything to do with them."

Meanwhile it appears that he has heard about the production unit that has been set up there, and this has attracted his attention. "It might be of advantage to us if they could supply us with vegetables, considering the long feeder lines that presently supply the castle," he says. He will see what the castle has to offer in return for the tomatoes. That would be a start. I will have to come to an arrangement with them.

And indeed, the transaction is successful and my first mission is thereby completed. Before long I shall no doubt be asked to do something else. However, when I look out across the sea I notice that this area is not as peaceful as I had thought. A ship is approaching that looks like a warship. I am not sure whether I really want to explore these images any further. It looks as if the people on the ship are Spanish and I don't like the look of them at all. There has been enough trouble with them in other parts of the world and no doubt they are now going to make a nuisance of themselves here.

The men step ashore and within moments there is a clattering of arms. A delegation makes its way to the commander, but apparently this results in nothing, because it then looks as if there is about to be a battle. They are demanding possession of the area, and a fight is therefore unavoidable.

Our dragon ship is bobbing on the waves nearby. The Viking captain had stayed in the neighborhood all the time. His ship can sail both on the sea and in the air. We are now busy pumping a huge tank full of water and when we have finished we rise into the air with our vessel. When we are above the warship we drop the tank of water. I see the tip of the mast piercing the tank, and so all their gunpowder gets wet in one go. For the moment we shall leave it at that.

Economics or Warfare

If for a moment we leave aside the pilfering from the cellars of the castle, then it appears that the main line of the story leads to the idea of development aid. A tomato surplus is produced and this provides the first bartering counter. In the past, tomatoes were a sign of fertility and love. This is no longer so in our materialistic age. Tomatoes are simply tomatoes, and that is why the captain wants to be in on it. He smells trade.

You feel slightly worried as you make your way toward him. If only there is no trouble brewing, you think. Well, it doesn't look too bad, he seems businesslike. I think it is not impossible that you have gone back on board ship at this point. Listen to what he is telling you. His argument is very interesting.

Up to now they had kept at a distance because there had been trouble in the past. (Presumably when they seized possession of the place and built their castle there!) Nor is it their policy to be aggressive. (Well, well.) And they had not had any intention of doing anything about those Indians. (But didn't you tell me they were very sick?) Now he has heard about a production unit that has been set up and therefore he thinks it is important that an official contract should be drawn up. (So that is how it is: people are not interesting in themselves, least of all when they are sick. They become interesting only when there is profit in it. Only then does it become feasible to use them in the economic process and make them subservient to it.)

The logical course for you now is to round off your mission and conclude a contract, which you succeed in doing.

Let us, before we go any further, make a little excursion into the mythology of horses, which is to be found all over the world. The horse was connected with the sun and with the king, and eventually, of course, with the sun king. The rites relating to the horse were war rites and came within the compass of a male-oriented order which, some thousand years before Christ, over-mastered the world of the mother goddess and of everything that is feminine. Coins in those days bore the image of a horse leaping over a bull. The bull was the symbol of the mother goddess earth and of the agrarian society, and this society is now being trampled underfoot by the cavalry.[21]

Something of this nature is now happening in your story about the palace. You are the protagonist in part of the history of mankind. You are standing at the beginning of a new era which will last more or less until the present day.

The end of that era is depicted in Picasso's *Guernica,* where we see a horse being brought down by the lance of its own rider. The bringers of light are no longer the sun and the moon, but the electric light bulb. The horse has been replaced by the horse power of aircraft and tanks.[22] Why do we need all those things to do with warfare? Surely the captain was not up to any mischief? Your second mission shows that there is something amiss in the situation at sea. A Spanish warship approaches, exactly at the moment when from a commercial point of view interesting developments are taking place.

You are not sure whether you wish to respond to these images, but it can't be helped. The feminine element is being subdued and the masculine element has quite different ideas. It wants to subject the entire world to itself, and does not mind a few bouts of fighting in order to get its way.

Women and children have helped to make the male into a hero figure. They have carefully educated him for the role, by depriving him of his emotions as far as possible. As a result he is not much plagued by uneasy feelings while the shooting takes place.

Soon enough it becomes obvious that you are not very clearly a "man." You nervously flee in the Viking's mother-ship. Never mind, you are still only an apprentice, and on board the ship you are able to think up a plan that is a match for the scorching power of the fire which is being ignited. Water has brought rescue here.

Have you noticed to what extent you were obliged to join in the game? You have to be able to justify warfare and that is why there must always be a white and black side. For convenience's sake the Spaniards have been made black in this case.

On their caps the cavalry men wear a circle with a cross in it. This sign occurs again and again in your story, whenever radical changes take place, or when something that is very precious has to be rescued or saved. In reality the same thing happens. Small wonder, therefore, that armies carry such a sign with them, in the hope that the gods will be on their side.

Last Sunday a well-known movie was shown on television portraying a similar situation at the time of the invasion of Normandy. The style was that of a Western. There were two sides: a group of heroes and a bunch of country yokels. The issue was a large hoard of gold. Live cartridges were used, as was clear from the outcome. Both sides wore a sign on their sleeve. The signs do not differ much from each other, in fact they are even almost identical. The myth in which you have become involved here is still alive.

The Hermit

We have decided to leave the castle domain and are now traveling in a northerly direction. Strangely, the sun is there too.

When we have arrived somewhere near the north pole I see a spit of land with a palm tree on it, which is of course impossible. How could that tree have found its way here, and how is it able to grow? There are enough questions here to make it worth while going ashore for further inspection.

When we reach the tree I see that there is a cave nearby with a man in it. He lives as a hermit and is clothed in animal skins. Yet he is not a savage. The cave contains all the things that are needed for one's daily life. The man is heating a kettle of water on a fire. He guards the tree and takes warm water to it every day. He must try to keep the tree alive, until circumstances change for the better and life has become possible in this desert.

The tree is kind of forerunner. The secret lies not only in the warm water. The man also has links with a star. I want to find out what his secret is. It is as if the man knows what is essential for life. Warmth is essential; so, it seems, is light. I see that the star is beamed at the man and not at the tree. He is linked with the cosmos, which puts him in possession of a certain kind of energy. I follow the man closely. The climate really seems to be changing. The south wind brings warmth. I am trying to find the connection, but I do not succeed.

Then I decide to ask the man about it. "Wait and see," he says, "it will become clear all by itself. Sit down and don't try to understand it." The star begins to shine, spreading a blue light. When we have sat in silence for a while, I notice that the light from the star has transferred itself to our eyes. I see two moving stalks of light in the man's eyes. Then I see the effect when you look at something. The plants begin to grow. The light has a life-giving quality, and it also brings health. A long time later I rise up on a cloud. In the distance I see mountain peaks sticking out above the clouds. On one of these there is a blue light. When you beam this at another mountain, you can take part in the life there. There is light on the other peaks as well. In this way it is possible to be in contact with everyone. There is also a woman who does not want to join in. In the air a kind of waferlike circle can be seen, with a crucifix pressed on it. I don't care much for this. The woman appears to be running away. When she turns, she aims a revolver and fires. The wafer falls into the crater of a volcano. Perhaps I am too high up to be able to continue, and had better return to the earth, and to the women's archipelago, which I have completely lost sight of.

The Idealist

You are sick and tired of it all, after that business with the castle, and you have moved away in the direction of the north pole. You have literally absconded, and all the signs point toward a new beginning. The road of blatant materialism turned out to be impassable. Man will perish on that road. You'd better not think, though, that your departure means that there will now be no more warfare at the castle. The fighting will carry on regardless, until the present day. So there is going to be a new beginning. After all that has happened, in the world of water and the world of fire, in this desert area, we shall now see the history of mother earth, and of how the earth became fertile.

It is the hermit in the cave who enables you to see what is to be done. The situation is so absured that you cannot fail to notice that the things that happen here are very strange. To assist a palm tree to grow by the north pole by means of a kettle of warm water—this really runs counter to all the rules. Your brain is therefore having to work overtime, because this is a phenomenon you had not reckoned with. Your attention is drawn by a bright star and by the light falling on the man. The south wind has to bring about a new climate, that is clear, but the most essential factor appears to come from the sky. That is where the light comes from which has to become fixed in our eyes. Don't attempt to understand it, says the hermit, sit down in it, in the light, then the change will occur all by itself.

Full of disbelief you do as you are told, because you have some awareness of cosmic energies and how they can penetrate into the world of matter. To your surprise you notice that you have begun to see differently. Before your eyes things begin to live and plants and animals begin to grow. You see the world flourish before your eyes. Once again you are involved in a mythical event. Listen for example to the story of the goddess Inanna in Mesopotamia. Her name means "goddess of the heavens" and she was called the first daughter of the moon, or the morning or evening star (the planet Venus). She was responsible for the growth of plants and animals and for the fertility of mankind.[23] On the clay tablets from that time we read the following: "At that time, in those very first days, one single tree, a huluppu tree [probably a palm tree] had been planted on the bank of the Euphrates. The south wind tugged at its roots and pulled at its branches until the waters of the Euphrates carried it away. Then I, Inanna, lifted the tree from the water and took it to my sacred garden and there I tended it."[24]

That it is possible to look at the reality around you in different ways, has become clear on several previous occasions. Without the spirit and without wonderment, everything seems flat. All things are ordinary and they do not inspire you to anything. You almost die of boredom and your life becomes hollow. To your amazement, on more than one occasion this same world showed a quite different face. From moment to moment you saw the snow, for example, in two different guises and you realized with a shock that it is possible to reduce life to a banal event.

You can try, then, to look at the small world in the little yard behind your house with different eyes, but the hermit has advised you against that. You won't succeed just by looking differently. It is a question of a very parodoxical event. You cannot organize the light, you can only sit down in it and then it will become clear all by itself. The rest must come from the other side, it will have to fall from the sky. Perhaps you can try to make yourself receptive to this.

Off you are again. After this lofty event you have gone straight into the air. With search lights you scan the sky and there you discover several fellow sufferers. It appears possible to take part in the life of others while being seated on your own mountain. High above everything and with your head in the clouds you

seem to be uniting the nations into a universal brotherhood of
men. But once again a whistle calls you back. Now a woman has
risen up inside you, to fire a shot at the cross in the circle. We did
not know that women were able to do this, but facts are facts, and
she is clearly aiming at something. Or perhaps she is aiming at
you. You threatened to become unfaithful to the earth and you
now realize that it is better to go down and resume the thread
there, if possible together with the woman of the archipelago.

Every ending of a series of imaginations is arbitrary. Now that
you have traveled through all the elements—water, fire, earth,
and air, we shall draw a conclusion. In this series you have so far
occupied yourself with a number of personal problems. But they
were not only personal problems. You were involved with the
troubles and difficulties of mankind as a whole. Strangely enough,
you were not asked to think about these world problems, even
though that had to be done. No, you became the leading actor in
a number of key moments in this great drama. In this way you
were able to try to find your own answers to the challenges that
have presented themselves in our civilization in the past and that
are still with us today. You have also done a bit of work for me by
taking part in this, for which I want to thank you most warmly.

This Time It Was My Turn

At the beginning of the imaginations I was faced with the
question "Who am I?" I was unable to get a grip on the
meaning of my existence. Time and again I had to try, with the
aid of my intelligence, to develop a more comprehensive vision,
but I did not succeed in bridging the insoluble contradictions.
First of all there was the dilemma of how to give a direction to
my life while at the same time being steered and determined
by my environment. In my relationship with a girlfriend I
experienced the same ambiguity: what do I myself want and
what am I allowing to be done to me. I was unable to solve the

problem, and when the relationship broke up I was in utter despair.

Initially the situation in my imaginations was chaotic. But at a certain moment I discovered that I did not need to accept all the images. I began to distinguish between meaningful and not meaningful images, and I learned how to choose between them.

At first the images were mostly concerned with motives, to which I dared not give free rein in my daily life. I became aware of the kind of fears and dark longings that were stirring in my mind. At times quite a lot of courage was needed to admit the images at all. In fact, I had often seen them long before, but there was such a taboo on them still that I dared not have anything to do with them. At such moments I was inclined to give myself instructions about what I was allowed to feel. Only gradually did I begin to realize that admitting unacceptable feelings did not in any way imply that I was at their mercy. I was still able to choose, and I could reject them if I wished. By far the most important thing was to face up to them, which enabled me to be actively engaged with the products of my unconscious. In this way a stronger link was formed between the various parts of myself and a certain measure of cooperation between these parts was also created.

So it came about one day that for many hours I was riding on a black horse, in rain and in the darkness of night, through a totally empty landscape. Even the ground was not visible; there was only the horse. I relived my loneliness from the time prior to this event. The horse and I had no one but each other, and I was touched by the animal's faithfulness. We returned to the inhabited world together.

In my imaginations there was often an element of violence and aggression. I was always very startled at cruel incidents such as, for instance, pigs being skinned alive. These incidents had a lot to do with sex, and the relationship between men and women in the imagination occupied me for a long time. To me, there was something mysterious about women, and I was afraid of them. I think that this was probably the reason why I went to try and wheedle their secret out of them. During that journey there was a kind of turning point. I stopped chasing after them and started going my own way. In reality, something rather similar happened. My life ceased to be dominated by this question.

The aggressive element has not altogether gone, but it has become less violent. It is as if a connection has been made with my curiosity, which means that I can direct my energy toward reaching certain goals, and that I can be more open to other people. It also means that I am able to think about certain things with a sense of humor and that I no longer cling so anxiously to all kinds of truths. I even found that there was now room for apparently useless things such as abandoning myself to rhythm in dance and music. By playing with colleagues I was able to clear my head and make myself open to others.

I think that my longing for the great, all-embracing absolute is in fact a spiritual longing, the wish to penetrate what lies outside our reality and to experience that our world is not purely external. It was important to me to throw aside predigested group-beliefs and to go in search of my own values.

It seems to me that the values in our culture have at times degenerated into a thin veneer. A quick wash by a few economic setbacks causes much of it to disappear, as if the values were based on little more than a bit of "social talk," on facades and moralistic twaddle.

A different kind of thinking was set in motion in me. The scientific, methodical thought is still present, but beside it I now have scope for the stream of thought to which you do not have to give any direction, and which allows new creativity to bud from old rigidity.

At the moment I am trying to create a life for myself in society as it is at present. Inevitably, I too shall have to submit to wage slavery. My main concern will be that I do not at the same time surrender myself as well. It is a precarious equilibrium. I have to keep telling myself that it is merely a game and that I should not take it too seriously. I must take care of myself and not allow myself to become dependent on a job or on the welfare state. I am beginning to feel just a little confident that I will find my way.

I am a man of extremes and many of my problems were a result of this. Time and again I lost sight of the opposite pole, and could no longer find the equilibrium. Again and again I saw contradictions, whereas in fact there are two poles between which a fruitful tension can exist. My discoveries are not really new, I know that, and yet it feels as though they are new. This has always been the case, but this time it was my turn to find out.

4 – PHENOMENA AND LAWS IN THE WORLD OF THE SELF

THE FORMATION OF IMAGINATIONS

THE INNER IMAGES

People live in two worlds at once, an inner and an outer world. Even the most outwardly directed people do so. Every now and then it is necessary to return to home base, even if only in order to prepare new measures for further action.

The border traffic between the two worlds runs very smoothly, so smoothly that at times it can no longer be said with certainty in which world we find ourselves: we wonder whether we have seen something for real or whether we have imagined it. The imaginal world we are dealing with here fulfills a number of important functions. One of these is the function of making preparations for the future. Our plans for the future can be tried out by means of inner imaginations, and if the trials turn out well we will carry out our plans in that way. In order to make our tests as realistic as possible, in certain cases we can make use of images from our memory, which can have a large degree of reliability. In other cases we shall have to create new images, because we do not know from experience what they look like. We visualize the new situation as clearly as possible and test our actions.

In this way it is possible to travel back and forth in time, so that we can be alternately in the past, the present, and the future. And we can move from one space to another, so that we can experience events in other parts of the world.

It has been known for some time that these inner images can

have a great influence on us. They can cause us to be in a particular mood or cause us to have a particular feeling; similarly, our thoughts can be directed by them. The "fantasy" that something is going to turn out badly may well have as a result that we never embark on it; we prefer to stay in the misery we know already.[1] Better to have a toothache than go to the dentist. On the other hand, however, the images can also help us, and with the aid of our imagination we may be able to rid ourselves of a great deal of trouble.[2] Fantasies or images are not quite the same as imaginations in the sense in which we use the word here. In order to bring about imaginations certain conditions must be met first.

CONDITIONS FOR THE FORMATION OF IMAGINATIONS

The main characteristic of imaginations is that we ourselves do not have full control of the imaginal situation and that in some cases we have no control over it at all.

Something enters from the other side which we had not expected. This may surprise or baffle us, it may move us emotionally or can arouse any other feelings in us; it can frighten us and even deter us.

The first condition for the formation of imaginations is that we begin to direct our concentrated attention to the world of inner images. It therefore requires in the first place a measure of concentration, and this is the reason why it bears some resemblance to certain forms of meditation. You have to close yourself off from the outer world for a while, and you must occupy yourself only with what goes on inside you. It is therefore advisable to close one's eyes during the imagination, although some people can see the inner images even when their eyes are open.

By means of concentration and of focusing the attention, we find that a number of things will happen at once. Certain figures will detach themselves from the background and very soon all kinds of associations will be set in motion in us, with the result that the world of images begins to acquire meaning. Sometimes several figures demand our attention simultaneously and then it is a question of choosing: am I going to occupy myself with this or with that? Directing our attention also leads us to feel involved with the imaginal figuration. It does something to us: it makes us curious, appeals to us, makes us experience something or arouses a certain aversion in us. In short, the images invite or repel, but in both cases we are inclined to begin to do something with them.

The second condition is that we allow the images to change spontaneously. It is chiefly because of these changes that events different from the ones we ourselves are programming can occur. In most cases the effect is very surprising. Images will appear on the screen that may lie far away from reality and so it may happen, for instance, that fairy-tale figures appear, or mythological characters, such as have been encountered by people throughout the centuries.

The non-realistic character of the images makes it necessary to interpret them. What does this or that image signify? What does it resemble? What thoughts and experiences does it arouse in me? As we attribute meanings, a problem occurs: things can no longer be defined unambiguously. We enter the world of parables and symbols and are faced with the realization that symbols can often express several things at once, and that our ordinary thought processes are inadequate to deal with this. As is known from the practice of meditation,[3] involuntary forces will then make their appearance in us, which appeal to a different part of our brain and our personality.

The third condition is the active involvement of the ego. This can happen in several different ways, firstly by tracking down the inner logic according to which the images are developed.[4] Why am I being confronted with this image and with this event? What am I to conclude from it? The fact that, for instance, the flowers in the garden let their heads droop when I feel sad, can be understood without further explanation. But what am I to think of the gardener who, without saying a word, hands me a little white flower? And what is the meaning of the little house which, apart from one small window, is completely under the ground? And if I do not know what to do with the flower, is it a coincidence that there happens to be a little cupboard with a lock in the wall? Could this perhaps be a hint?

There is an inner logic at play, although it is not always easy to track it down. There doesn't seem to be much cooperation in this respect. The unconscious Self can let us go on struggling on our own for a long time, without in any way facilitating our task. The only thing that usually proceeds unhindered is the constant changing of the images. Different pictures and situations keep appearing, which may lead to a gradual improvement in clarity.

A second form of involvement, which is directly linked to the first, concerns *taking action*. We saw it in the example of the garden: it is possible to go for a walk in that garden. It's ten to one that at the beginning of the imagination we find ourselves standing on a path and we may safely assume that the path leads somewhere. If you can't immediately find anything to do, you might do worse than take a walk, and wait to see what you meet and what happens. In this way, too, changes keep occurring in the place of action.

The third form of involvement is that of *interaction*. You can make contact with the different figures and when you have become used to the situation it is quite normal to start up a conversation with the people you meet.

So it can happen that when you are in the little house, the gardener passes by after a while. And when you ask him, "What have you come for?" it may be that he says, much to your amazement, "I have come to get my flower back, because you are not looking after it properly. It isn't getting enough fresh air and you don't give it enough compost," until you understand that he is really talking about you.

OUR ATTITUDE TOWARD THE IMAGINAL PICTURES

It is not at all self-evident that a person will want to be involved with his imaginations. It is important to examine our attitude toward the unconscious Self. In our civilization today we have become so used to acknowledging only the existence of an ego that it may be difficult to find a satisfactory attitude toward those images in which the unconscious Self manifests itself. It can happen that the ego and the Self operate in two quite different directions and that no useful contact can be achieved. It is important to bring about sound interplay at the beginning of a series of imagination.

Let us make this clear with an example: suppose you don't have much confidence in your own strength. As long as life is sunny, all goes well, but as soon as a frightening situation occurs things go wrong. Suppose that during your imagination you find yourself in a sea and that you are floating pleasantly on the blue water. Suddenly, something begins to pull you down and then you feel anxiety. What should you do at such a moment? Do you still have the confidence that these images can do no harm? If you don't, you will probably drop out. You open your eyes and the whole frightening situation has gone. You assume that the unconscious Self is not to be trusted. Or in simple language, you no longer trust yourself.

How do people manage to gain experience in dealing with frightening images and to be at ease with themselves? Listen to someone's own words:

> I am floating in the sea and see something black moving about in the water. I am being dragged down by my hair. I turn around and look into the water to see who is doing this to me. Within seconds there is a fight. There is a snakelike animal down there, very eerie, and pitch-black. I can't put up with that kind of thing. I ask the animal who sent him. He points at a Jesuslike figure on the beach. "What's the meaning of this," I call out. "I sent him to make you stronger," he replies. I say, "I wish we had come to the point when I don't need that kind of thing any longer." He laughs and calls out, "You've come a long way already; as soon as you have overcome those negative feelings about yourself you will have reached your goal. And it is already obvious that you have enough strength."

The woman who says these words is making a totally intuitive distinction between what the scary beast does (his behavior) and what the behavior signifies.[5] She clearly assumes that the snake's frightening actions have a purpose—stronger still, that the purpose is a positive one. Unfortunately, this unpleasant activity is still necessary at this moment, but perhaps it will soon no longer be necessary; once she has become strong enough the snake will be allowed to disappear. The positive attitude which is here adopted with regard to the unconscious Self is decisive for further growth.

The Second Center Beside the Ego

THE INITIATIVES OF THE UNCONSCIOUS SELF

There are two ways in which we can enter our imaginal world. The first is very clearly directed toward a specific aim, because we want to see something specific, the sea for instance, and sure enough, if that is what you have in mind, the sea will indeed appear. The other way is to let anything occur at random. In that case you may find yourself in a world which you would never have dreamed of, so that you need to look around carefully for a while in order to find out where in heaven's name you are.

In both cases, however, the unconscious Self is present in the imaginal situation. You may be by the sea, but why are there for instance no other people, and why does a boat suddenly sink below the waves? Apart from the things we actually seek, we may also be faced with aspects of the things with which we are unconsciously preoccupied. That is why we must all the time ask the question: "What does this situation have to tell me and what can be its purpose?"

THE OFFERED SITUATION

The situation as it is offered in the images impresses a mark on the person who enters it. This is clear as soon as something appears that has a strong appeal to us. When this happens, you may respond by lying down to bask happily in the sun or you plod laboriously through the soft sand. Sometimes the expectation that something is about to happen can be deceptive. For what are you to think of a landscape in which there is nothing or nobody to be seen? You wander on and on and for fifteen minutes or more nothing happens at all.

In such cases you may be inclined to think that the rule does not apply to you. Or perhaps the contrary is true, perhaps you are completely determined by the situation. You show so little initiative yourself that the course of events remains utterly monotonous. This can happen especially when you have been taught systematically that you should not take action on your own behalf, or when you yourself have chosen to play such a role. It is then of the utmost importance to break the power of the situation.

Every offered situation has a number of typical characteristics that can provide us with information about the problems which at that moment play a role in our life. For example, every landscape has a specific symbolic force.[6] Entering a damp cave suggests a different theme from walking up a path leading to a mountain top. The landscape points to a particular inner mood and offers the possibility of opening up specific problem areas.

ROADS AND CROSSROADS

We have already mentioned that every road leads somewhere and can therefore be used as an invitation to set off toward a goal. If the road is straight and immensely long so that the end is not in sight, there is little reason to expect anything new. If there is anything to see, you can usually see all there is at a glance, right from the start. But if you are out for adventure, you will probably find yourself at the beginning of a winding path with unsuspected twists at the end of the journey. Thus the mere presentation of various situations and the kinds of paths and roads can suggest that there is a hidden intention behind the images we see. Almost invariably, the intention is to get us to act. If this is not successful, or if we are too passive, then a crossroad may appear before our eyes, so that our ability to choose is put to the test. There is no

signpost. Often there is some indication to suggest what difference it will make which road we choose. One road leads to the
sea, another to a wood and the third leads to the inhabited world.
You can choose whichever one you want.

The unconscious Self does not always take charge of the situation, especially when you are still too undecided yourself. Once
you have made up your mind and are prepared to follow the sug-
gestions, the initiative of the Self can take on impressive forms.[7]
We might also say that you have to believe in its power, which is
probably true of all therapies.

THE GUIDES

On our journey we can meet all kinds of creatures that demand
our attention. This is particularly true of those creatures which
we shall call the guides. They are usually animals which have been
placed there deliberately to show us the way. In the preceding
therapies there are several examples of this. The guide does not
usually speak, but indicates by means of gestures that he is not
there for nothing. It may be a duck, quacking vociferously and
pointing with his beak to his back, as a signal for you to sit down.
Or it may be a rabbit, putting a carriage in front of you and indicating with his paw that you should get into it. Sometimes the
animal uses actual words: "Why are you standing there, looking
at the eclipse of the sun, do you want me to take you to the sun?"

Once you have become used to taking the advice of these guides,
you will notice how much benefit this can bring. The place where
the guide takes you will turn out to be well worth studying.

Dealing with imaginal situations, roads, and guides arouses a
particular ability in us, that of unconscious knowledge or intuition.[8] Things are not made known explicitly and yet you simply
know what is intended. You also know that you can safely go up
in the air on the back of the duck and that you are in no danger of
falling off. And if you did fall off, you can still be sure that once
down on the ground you will stand up and look around you in
order to find out what was the meaning of such rough treatment.

Should you land in such a savage world and yet not lose your faith, you will be rewarded.

THE OPPOSING PLAYERS

They provide the opposition and it is their aim to *set the inner dynamics in motion* and to *make development possible in situations of stagnation or regression.*

Often the guide will point the way to the opponent: for example, the horse takes you to the princess and the rabbit has placed a carriage in front of you in order to take you to a fisherman. Both are there to provide interplay: the princess by inviting you to give a reception together with her. She lets you shake hands with people and you have no idea why. But it arouses a lot of questions in you. So does the fisherman, because he is fishing for icicles which then lie melting on the bank. This makes you think about questions that lie far beyond your horizon.

Probably this need for counterplay is the reason why the opposing players are often of the opposite sex. The inner dynamics are set in motion by means of polarities, and the stagnation seems to have occurred because of a fixation on one of the two poles.[9]

The unconscious Self finds the necessary players and often provides a challenging opposition, but it does not create the game itself. You have to develop the game, and much depends therefore on the question whether or not you are prepared to respond to the challenges. If ideas come to your mind and you carry them out, then the opponents are sure to respond. The most important thing is that you find the beginning. Usually we operate in the first instance with experiences from our childhood as our starting point, when our parents were still the opposite players. These experiences form a matrix for what you will expect later in the imaginations. However, the opposing players often do something different from what you expected, and it can even happen that ideal parents appear, so that you simply have no idea any longer what is going on. If your confidence in your real parents has been greatly damaged, it will be very difficult to muster enough confidence with regard to these new players, who are acting so differently. On the other hand, it is equally difficult to remain systematically mistrustful, and it is therefore possible that much damage from the past may be repaired. As long as you receive often enough what you were deprived of in the past and for which you have been longing ever since, the ice can melt for you too, and a positive development can be brought about.

The opponent may have a great deal to put up with, as the following example will show. "In front of me stands a black bird with a yellow beak. He is picking at his feathers and is completely turned in upon himself. I hate that kind of behavior. However much I implore and bet, he does not react. Then I give him a push so that he falls to bits on the ground. His head goes on looking at me, with one eye. I am sorry for what I have done and start stroking his head gently. Then the whole bird starts to grow together again, starting from the head, and he says, 'You should not have done that.'"

THE CORE FIGURES

When we look at the figures in the imaginations we get the strong impression that there is a central organization. It is for this reason that in the introduction we spoke of the core of the Self. We are not in a position to expand further on this. In the imagination of the talisman in Chapter 2 there occurs the figure of a gardener. He has an ordinance survey map with him on which all areas from previous imaginations occur. The only place that is not shown on it is the place on which the man is standing at the moment; that place is shown on the back of the map. This indicates something about a "reality" which is different from ordinary reality. You could say reality has a front and a back. The back of reality is not subject to the laws of finite time. Hence the fact that he calls himself the Eternal One and Life.

It seems that this core figure has the management of a whole series of imaginations.[10] He is the director, but from time to time he is also a player, as appears from the imagination about the old

man and the sketch book in Chapter 1. Here too we encounter a
person who occurs in the imaginal reality but who at the same
time stands above and outside it, which means that he can become an anchorage providing a firm hold in times of uncertainty.

A role closely related to that played by the Eternal One is
played by various divine figures that appear from time to time, for
instance, when the woman sees the following:

> I am floating in the water of the sea. The sun (again the sun)
> goes down behind the palm trees. On the horizon I see a calm
> figure, a sort of woman with several arms and with her legs
> folded under her. She radiates calm, a calm strength. She beck-
> ons to me. I detach myself from the water and feel that I must
> approach her with respect. I feel awe. There is a red cushion on
> which I can sit. When I look into her eyes I almost feel sick with
> emotion. She has a sad expression, but it is not personal. It is
> more a question of a collective grief which she carries within her.
> "Yes," says the woman, "weeping goes further than crying. You
> weep and that is good. Allow yourself to weep." She strokes my
> feet and this feels very gentle. "Yes," she says, "gentleness and
> weeping belong together; it is good that you have come."
>
> Between her eyes I see a beautiful shape with crystal stars. I
> ask her what this means. She replies, "You will learn to under-
> stand. It is still too early. As long as you leave the sea often
> enough."

Here again is a core figure who knows what is hidden behind
the visible things. The multiple arms are reminiscent of an Indian
goddess. She inspires great awe. It must be noted, however, that
her presence points to developments that cannot be forced. They
require time, and they also demand that the ego choose such a
development in complete freedom.

Our Inner World Is a World Apart

THE WORLD IMAGE IN IMAGINATIONS

There is a need to say something about the world image in imaginations. This need follows from the fact that phenomena occur in

imaginations that are not known in the outside world. One such phenomenon is that life in the imaginal inner world takes place not only on earth but also in the sky and in the water, or rather, under the water and even under the ground. You might say that the imaginations operate with a very ancient world image, in which the universe is divided into a heaven, an earth, and an underworld.

Heaven. It is always good to be in heaven. When you are there you are temporarily withdrawn from the hurly burly down below. You can float around to your heart's delight, there is always a suitable cloud on which you can nestle to take a rest. This gives you the opportunity to observe a certain distance and relativity, which enables you to come to some conclusions about what is to be done next.

It is easy to move about in the sky: you can hover on your own, but there is also a large assortment of flying creatures offering their services as flying taxis. All of a sudden a bird stands before you, inviting you for a trip on his back, or you are being fitted with wings of your own, so that you can fly by yourself. If need be there is an angel near by to show you the way.

If you find it difficult to take initiatives on your own, there are other ways. For instance, a whirlwind may come to your aid and exercise so much suction power that you cannot help going up in the air—or, rather, it makes you want to go up in the air. You are being whisked around numerous times and then, gently or not so gently, you are dropped somewhere. When you land, you will have lost your bearings for a moment, for you have arrived in a new part of your inner world, or at any rate in an area where you do not come very often. There is no doubt that it is very important to have a good look around.

Earth. On earth many things take place in the manner to which we are accustomed, with the difference that accidents are not fatal in the usual way. For instance, you can crash into a tree and yet stay alive. You can be threatened by a tiger and simply remark,

"There is a furious tiger standing before me, exactly in the place where I want to be. What might he want? Maybe he is going to eat me, but I know that if he does I will simply go on living. Let me see why he is so angry. He says he is angry because he is locked up. I know that feeling. I suggest to him that we look for a solution together, and he agrees." If the man had decided to chase the tiger, the outcome would no doubt have been different and he might well have been eaten up.

A tiger does not appear for no good reason. The aggression of the animal was obviously related to the aggression of the imaginator. Being afraid of a tiger means, therefore, being afraid of your own aggression. To conquer this fear means that a new road is cleared, namely the possibility of tackling the badness inside you.

In brief, these images occur in order that you may make progress within yourself. For instance, suppose the ground suddenly begins to crumble away under your feet. This can happen on the edge of a ravine, and if you can't quickly find something to hold on to, you topple into the abyss together with a lot of chunks of rock. Once you have gotten over your fright, you get up and walk on. A useful question to ask is this: why did that rock crumble? You can be sure it did not crumble for no reason. Was there perhaps a moment of panic? A flash in which you thought you were losing control, up there on the edge? That would be enough to be translated into an image, and down you go. If you should find yourself in a similar situation again and you succeed in subduing your panic in good time, there may be a few little stones rolling down, but that is all. Peace returns and you can carry on as usual. Moreover, the panic will not come back so easily after that. You may have to struggle for a while, but you must be prepared to accept that, if the panic is to disappear from your daily life.

The Underworld. There are many roads leading to the underworld. When swimming, you sometimes notice that you are being pulled down or that you are being sucked to the bottom by a whirlpool. Sometimes people simply walk into the sea and continue their way on the bottom of the ocean. Quite often there will be a shipwreck that you can enter, and there will be a hatch somewhere, giving access to an underground passageway. In the earth there are also entrances to the underworld. Sometimes these are through a manhole cover and sometimes through a little door in a tree. You step inside and find stairs leading down. Sometimes you get to the underworld through a cave or by straying into a marsh and sinking into the mire. Of course this is not very pleasant but at least you stay alive. After a number of these disagreeable experiences you begin to discover why these things happen. Or you don't understand it, but without realizing it you have nevertheless come to adopt a different pattern of behavior and to have different feelings. The images change whether you understand the situation or not. You don't need to understand everything in order to undergo a favorable development. You respond unconsciously.

One notorious entrance to the underworld is the black hole. In certain cases this is the first image people see and they are often faced with a "black hole" in real life as well. When you look into the black hole for a long time you will notice that something begins to change. You will notice that you can go down into it and land somewhere and yet stay alive.

THE SUN AND THE MOON

The sun and the moon represent a polarity; that is, they are connected with each other while at the same time there is a contrast between them. In imaginations this may be demonstrated, for instance, by women seeing a sun and men seeing a moon. The sun and the moon are then representations of the opposite poles. People are usually to a large extent unaware of their opposite pole, but when the sun or the moon appears as an antipole in an image, this appearance often forms the beginning of a process of growing awareness. A good example of this can be found in Chapter 3 of this book, where there is talk of a "new phase" for people. In that particular imagination the influence of the moon increases greatly; that is, the unconscious forces rise to the surface.

If the sun suddenly becomes very important to a man, then we can speak of a further development of the masculine identity. Sun and moon can appear in their true form, but it is also possible that instead of the moon an image appears of the moon goddess or of water—the element that is her domain. If the sun is to be represented, then the sun god may appear or the element that belongs to him, fire. In the following extract we find an example of this.

I feel as if I am still not regarded as fully fledged. When I am with my contemporaries I have the impression that they have made the grade and that I have not even begun. I want to do something about this in the images.

I see a sun god or a sun king, something like that. He is seated on a litter which is carried by many people. I am standing by the side. He sees me and says, "I am here for you too." In one hand he is holding a decorated staff and in the other a golden spoon. I decided to speak to him. I say that I have seen him before and ask whether he can perhaps help me to get ahead in the world. He is wearing a large feather headdress and in front of him he is holding a large round shield. "Certainly," he says, "I have seen you before too, and I can help you, because you are a son of the people." Then he pulls two feathers out of his headdress, dips the points into a fire and gives them to me. I have to draw something with these feathers. With my right hand I draw, completely automatically, an open hand and with my left hand I draw a fist.

He takes both these hands and brings them toward each other. They have to hold each other. It causes hurt and grief. One of the hands is in a stiff cramp and squeezes the other hand until it almost breaks. He puts a coin into the left hand and then it opens. I say, "It would be good if these two hands trusted each other." He asks me what is the matter with that left hand. I say, "It looks like a claw" and when I look at it I see it is a tiger's claw. I stroke the tiger on the head and he walks away into the desert.

I ask, "What should I do in order to become more relaxed?" He says, "Follow the tiger. He will be able to help you."

This is what happens when a man meets the sun god. He is addressed as a son of the people. Exactly the opposite happens in

Chapter 2 of this book. The woman in question can tell from the state of the water (the domain of the moon goddess) what her own situation is like. The water is frozen and there are icicles in the stream. The sun is needed here as an opposite pole, and the fisherman shows how it becomes possible for the sunlight to penetrate into the water. The real breakthrough occurs when the fire is brought in to melt the ice. The two poles of sun and moon must keep each other in equilibrium.

THE ELEMENTS AND THE FOUR WINDS

The Chinese knew about the elements in very early times. Later the ancient Greeks thought about them, and theories about the elements spread also to the rest of Europe. The Native Americans knew about them and so did the peoples of Africa and India. The elements represent certain forces in the imaginal inner world of man. They constitute its basic data.[11]

In the examples I have cited, these data appear again and again. The symbolic force of the elements and their connection with, for instance, the winds, is varied and complex. In the West, the theory of elements was abandoned long ago, but it might be worthwhile to take a fresh look at it, through a study of dream symbolism and of the data obtained from the imaginal world.

In our examples information about the elements crops up, especially in Chapter 3, where the man in question makes a cosmic journey and travels to the four winds where he comes in contact with the various elements. There seems to be an organized cohesion, but it is not yet clear how the connections are to be made.

In the therapy described in Chapter 3 it is demonstrated that each of the various elements can exercise its own influence on the person, and how the person will develop further seems to depend on the relationship between these influences.

THE ACCOMPANIMENT OF IMAGINATIONS

Not everyone needs to be accompanied by a therapist when working with imaginations. In principle, it is possible to do everything oneself. In practice, however, many people, especially at the beginning, prefer to receive support, for a variety of reasons:

- Your thoughts will often lead you to places other than those where the images occur. The therapist can help you not to wander off.
- "Scary" things may occur that frighten you and make you wonder whether they really belong to the imagination. When this happens it is important that there is someone near you who has witnessed such terrors before and knows that they do not last for long and that when they are gone the world will look different again. Such a person will be able to say to you, "If you are brave enough, wait and see what happens next and try to find out what is the meaning of it all."
- To many people it is important to be able to put their experiences into words at the moment that they have them. This sharpens their attentiveness and makes them more alert to what is significant. Putting things into words is a first step toward taking action. You do not merely undergo something but you also *do* something.

The therapist who accompanies the imaginations must therefore serve various purposes.

EFFECTIVE IMAGINATIONS

The therapist's first purpose is to bring about an effective imagination, that is to say, to make sure that three necessary conditions are met: (1) the subject must experience an imaginal world; (2) the images must be allowed to change spontaneously; (3) the subject must become actively involved in the imaginal world.

In order to achieve all these things it is useful to ask certain questions, such as the following.

- What do you see or what do you experience?
- Where exactly are you and what are you doing?
- What happens there? Is anything changing?
- Can you talk to the figure you see?

The relationship between the therapist and the imaginator is a very special one. In order to carry out his (or her) task, the therapist is completely dependent on the information he receives from the person who is being accompanied. In order to form an idea of the place of action and of the images that occur, he must be kept up to date from moment to moment. All that is available to him is "radio contact." He is told things by someone who is extremely busy and who keeps his ground station informed as he goes along, perhaps asking for further instruction from time to time, because he is in a situation reminiscent of some monstrosity on the moon. It is all utterly strange to him. By means of all his senses the imaginator perceives an unfamiliar world and wishes to know what other people who have been there have experienced and what he can and cannot permit himself to do there. This is why two people set off on the journey together and must try to interact with each other as well as they possibly can.

PROBLEM SELECTIVITY

The therapist's second purpose is to see that the subject makes progress with finding a solution to a problem. In a sense this is a false purpose. Imaginations do not necessarily have to be used for solving your problems. At moments when you don't have any problems it can be a happy experience to enter the imaginal world. Even then it remains a challenging world, which can be an inspiration in many ways. Many creative and artistic achievements have found their beginnings in this way. If, however, you are in a muddle with yourself, then the encounter between the ego and the Self can acquire the very special purpose of trying to get out of the difficulties. The accompaniment will then be directed toward this aim. Imaginations cannot in themselves get you out of trouble. You can try to exploit the possibilities of your imaginal world and use them for your particular purpose, and the therapist will keep a close eye on whatever information is given by the Self. In that case it will be important to pay close attention to the actions and reactions of the Self insofar as they are related to the specific problem situation you are in. It will then appear that the Self can provide an extensive range of learning situations that may be of help in solving the problems. The therapist may assume that the imaginator's ego has already tried everything possible to find a solution.

We can therefore direct our attention to the contributions made by the Self. How can the situations be evaluated from that perspective? Let us take the example of the dwarf and the strawberry plant from Chapter 1 of this book.

- First, we find that the imaginator's ego is busy trying to influence the situation in a positive way. (The dwarf waters the strawberry plant.)
- Second, the odds are too great. (The witch proves capable of threatening not only the strawberry plant but also the dwarf.)
- Third, there is a skeleton that can be brought to life, so that a knight is created who is able to turn the tide.

In this situation it is necessary that the imaginator see himself not only as the dwarf but realize that he can also become the knight. The therapist's role must in such cases be aimed at following the Self in its efforts. The imaginator must know that there is a knight hiding inside him and that he can use this knight to make the threats go away. The Self has shown that there is knightly courage present, even though it has yet to be awakened. In some cases it is necessary for the subject to be made aware of this possibility. In the course of the imaginations a new threat may occur, as happened a little while later in this same example.

On his way to the church the man meets two devils by the entrance; at such a moment it is important to know that a knight is not afraid of devils. The therapist's questions "What are you going to do about those devils?" is answered with "I get angry and I start to hit out at them. I raise hell and I smash them to bits."

In this way the ego receives support in its precarious situation and part of the problem is solved. At the same time, however, something else becomes clear as well.

THERAPEUTIC ACTIONS

The Self has at its disposal a fabulous repertoire of healing or, if you like, *therapeutic actions*. Of course, as a therapist one can seize on these imaginations in order to start a therapy of one's own. This can be a splendid idea, if the therapist has the necessary skills to do so. If one doesn't, or if one wants to learn more first, then it is advisable to let the Master (i.e., the Self) go his own way and not get under his feet. It is quite likely that after a while you will decide always to cede priority. If that is your choice: to give priority to the actions of the Self, then this does not mean that the therapist has lost his function from then on. However forceful the interventions of the Self may be, nothing will be undertaken unless the ego wishes it and gives it full cooperation. The ego retains its total freedom and the Self, however impressive its manifestation may be, will modestly withdraw as soon as the ego no longer requires its assistance.

What can happen is that the ego does not exactly know in what way the Self might be of use, and sometimes, in very precarious circumstances, cannot even manage to ask the right kind of question. At such moments the therapist may intervene. For instance: "Do you think you could tell this woman who lives all by herself in the mountains something about your problems? Do you think she might have some idea what you could do?"

BOUNDARIES AND LIMITATIONS

My aim in the preceding passage was to show how the Self operates in imaginations, and I did so by emphasizing two things:

1. The Self operates according to an organized pattern.
2. The Self operates in a wide variety of creative forms.

These two factors together might create the impression that a solution now exists to all problems. Unfortunately, this is not the case. The first limitation is that not everyone is capable of producing imaginations. It is not yet sufficiently understood why this is so. The second limitation is that not all imaginations are equally forceful in their effects. Here again, we do not know precisely what factors play a role in this.

A third limitation is that not all problems are amenable to

being approached by means of imaginations. Since it is not my intention here to produce a manual for those who want to accompany imaginations, I will confine myself at this point to a reference to other literature.[12] Looking back at the preceding imaginations, we can make a number of observations regarding their boundaries. To accompany someone in an imagination can be compared with accompanying an astronaut by means of radio contact. That situation is also subject to boundaries: the contact must not be broken. You as the accompanist must remain up to date with the conditions in which the imaginator finds himself, and the latter must continue to respond to your instructions. If this is not done, nothing can be accompanied and it is better to stop altogether. Both, then, have a demanding task. For example, the imaginator must not surrender control, for that would make him the plaything of the events in the imaginations. This usually happens when the imaginator's anxiety becomes overwhelming, or when he does things only because he thinks that it will meet with the approval of the therapist, so that he leaves undone the things he himself would like to do. We shall speak further of anxiety later on. For the moment it suffices to mention the golden rule that anxiety is there to be banished, or, as one of the wise guides from the imaginations remarked: "We are going to eradicate this anxiety, root and branch." It is obvious, therefore, that anxiety must not be allowed to gain ground.

A second boundary is determined by the interest of the imaginator. His interest is the one and only thing that matters in the accompaniment to an imagination. The therapist must never be out to score successes, because that would doom the imagination to be lost in the mist.

THE INTERACTION BETWEEN ACCOMPANIST AND IMAGINATOR

In order to give an impression of such interaction in an actual case, I reproduce here an account of an imagination in which the participation of the accompanist is included. In the following dialogue, *A* stands for accompanist and *I* for imaginator.

A. Suppose you were allowed to choose a landscape that fits your situation at this moment, what kind of landscape would that be?

I. I would go to the beach, because my nerves are all on edge, and then I feel best on the beach.

A. Okay, then I have a suggestion to make. We can't go there for real, but I can help you to go there in your imagination. Would you like that?

I. Yes, I would.

A. These things usually work best if you close your eyes and then try if you can see the beach.

I. That seems funny to me. I don't know if that will work.

A. Well, it doesn't really matter. You can put your hands in front of your eyes if you prefer, and then concentrate on what you see. That is the main thing. First try to think of the beach and as soon as you see anything you tell me. . . . . Is anything happening yet?

I. Yes, I can see a beach. It is completely empty.

A. Fine. Well, you take a good look around first. . . . How do you feel about that, that the beach is empty?

I. I don't mind. I'd like to have a little house here.

A. Maybe you can make one come? . . . Have you done it?

I. Yes, it came at once. It's very small and it's built into the sand dunes on three sides. The only windows are on the side of the sea. The sun comes from behind.

A. Where are you at this moment?

I. I am inside the house. It's quite safe in there, but very dark.

A. Maybe you can do something about that?

I. There's no sun coming in here. I'd like to make it look cosy. Maybe it would look nice if I used shells, if the light fell on them. I want to go to the sea.

A. What's it like there at the moment?

I. It's warm and I want to get to the water. But I daren't go in. I'm sitting down by the edge of the water now.

A. What are you thinking about while you are sitting there?

I. That nothing is going to happen as long as I do nothing. I'd like to talk to somebody.

A. Are there any other people on the beach now?

I. Yes, there are some, but I daren't talk to them.

A. Have a good look at them first. Maybe there is somebody among them who would be only too glad to talk.

I. The people I see don't have any faces.

A. No, that's right, people you don't know don't have faces for you yet. Is there anyone there that strikes you in particular?

I. There is someone in a black coat. It is an old man with a weather-beaten face.

A. Has he seen you?

I. Yes, he is looking at me because I am looking at him. It's as if he recognized me.

A. Do you think you could talk to him?

I. Yes, I think I might be able to. . . . (makes a gesture of surprise)

A. Is anything the matter?

I. He is taking his black coat off. He is dressed all in white now and he is coming toward me. He's sat down a little distance away from me, also by the edge of the water. There is nothing strange about it. It isn't frightening.

A. What is he doing?

I. He is looking at the horizon. And I am looking at him all the time. I daren't look at my shells any more now, because I am afraid he might go away then.

A. Can you tell him that?

I. He says, "I'll stay as long as I like."

I think that is a very hard answer. Now he's asking me what I am looking at all the time. I say I am looking at the shells. He can't see them and he comes closer to me. He likes them. I tell him I want to take them home with me. And I explain that I want to put them down there, so that they will give a bit of light. When he asks me where, I show him where the house is. He thinks it is funny that I want to take away these shells with me, when my house is so near by. You can see them here any day, he says. Then I tell him about my house and that it is so dark inside. And that I have been feeling so awful all along. He offers to help me. I am glad of that, but it also worries me.

Maybe I prefer to be alone for a while. He knows what I am thinking, it seems. He says, "If you want anything, just say." I ask, "But where will I be able to find you?" He answers, "I am always around here. If you want to see me, I am here."

A. Then maybe you can say goodbye to him now.

Some Learning Principles

In the imaginal world, learning does not in the first place consist of imprinting on your memory what you want to remember, nor in the analysis and logical construction of thought processes. The left half of our brain, which usually occupies itself so busily with such things, takes second place in the imaginal world. It is the other half that becomes active here.[13] A different aspect of our personality comes to the fore, and new qualities get a chance to develop. With the help of examples, we shall now describe and explain a number of learning principles that play a part in the imaginations.

LEARNING TO HAVE CONFIDENCE

By learning to have confidence we mean learning to have confidence in the Self. Although we normally talk of having or lacking self-confidence, and of confidence being able to grow, we do not usually practice learning to have confidence in the Self in any systematic way. In imaginations, however, you can't make much headway if there is a shortcoming in this respect. That is why it is usually the very first problem to be tackled.

From moment to moment an appeal is made to our willingness to self-surrender and active decision taking, without our having any clear idea where we are going or whether we will come back unscathed. Some people have a chance to build up their confidence gradually. They find themselves on a road which, to their surprise, really leads somewhere or they see an arrow pointing to somewhere. In other cases the previously mentioned guide may appear and take you somewhere.

But on what basis do we assume that we can safely take the
risk of starting the journey at all? In the best instances, we experience a special kind of radiance, which makes it easier for us to
gain confidence. The confidence itself will have to grow. It is not
so much a case of saying that you are confident as of doing something that proves you are confident. In the example of the encounter with the man in the black coat it can be clearly seen how
this works. Is there much reason to trust this man? His black coat
is not a particularly cheerful piece of evidence. More meaningful
might be his face. It is old and weather-beaten and bears a friendly
smile. The ego and the Self recognize each other.

All this is not enough, though, for the man does nothing as
long as no actual step is taken. The ego has to seek a rapprochement by demonstrating that it wishes to make contact. And then
the black coat slides down. This is the reply the man gives, and
the woman is vindicated in having given him her confidence.

THE CONFIRMATION

The Self replies by a confirmation: You have trusted me even
though I did not make it easy for you in my black coat, and by
doing so you have taken a very important step. In order to under-
line this and reinforce this strength in you, I take off my coat and
by appearing completely dressed in white I show you that I am
indeed to be trusted. The strength of the ego is reinforced so that
it can freely enter into communion with the Self. The woman now
makes a second discovery: having made contact she does not dare
break it again, because she is afraid the man will leave. When she
indicates this to him (another step taken), he replies, "I'll stay as
long as I like." In other words: the Self has a freedom of its own.
The woman can continue to look at the shells and do whatever
she wants to do without feeling afraid. Anxiety is not rewarded,
on the contrary, it is tackled with firmness. The reply therefore
hits hard.

"I'll stay as long as I like" does not mean "I am not interested
in you." In order to make this clear, he asks her what she is look-

ing at and he comes a bit closer in order to see better. The rapprochement comes from both sides.

Once the process of rapprochement between the ego and the Self has gotten under way, the therapist accompanying the imagination can take a step back. He needs to intervene only if something stagnates. In the example we have described it all runs smoothly.

The woman begins to talk about her house and in the language of these images this means: she is saying something about her situation and what she is up against. It is the language of parables: my situation can be known by the particulars of this house. The wise man, for there is no doubt that it is he, understands the message: "I am going through a terrible time and I badly want a bit of help, but I also want to keep my freedom. I would like you to come and help me by bringing some light and cheerfulness into my house down there, but when I want to be alone I want to be sure I can get rid of you again."

The answer is as simple as it is effective: "I am available whenever you call me," you might say. "I am prepared to help you, but then you will have to call me yourself, otherwise I will go my own way. You needn't fear that you won't be able to find me, because any moment you want to find me, and at any place, I shall be there. And when you have had enough of me I will disappear again."

THE TRIAL

The relationship between the ego and the Self has to be mutual. The ego will want to know where it stands, and as we saw just now, the Self leaves it in no doubt: "I am always near." The Self in its turn will want to know what the ego is prepared to do. This need not be more than what can be reasonably offered, but it must certainly be reasonable. A situation is planned in which both the Self and the ego can demonstrate how much can be relied on. A trial takes place, as we see in the following example.

The imaginator has a strong dislike of anyone who wants to

exercise power over her and she in her turn hates bossing anyone
else around. This kind of problem can also occur between the ego
and the Self, with the result that a barrier arises between the two.
The trial went as follows:

> There are stairs leading up, and at the top is a throne, a royal
> chair. Two very large lions lie there, one on each side of the
> throne. A red carpet leads to the throne. Meanwhile my mind is
> being terribly distracted by a fierce pain on the right side of my
> body. For the rest I can't see anything whatsoever, I only feel
> the pain. I believe I have an appointment here, but there is no
> one about. The pain is so bad that it drives me to seek advice
> from the lions. The lion on the right gives me a hard look. He
> clearly knows something about it and when I ask him he says,
> "Yes, I knew this was coming." Then I ask, "Do you also know
> by any chance who is causing me this pain?" The lion replies,
> "You are doing it yourself." Then I ask him whether something
> can be done about it and whether he can give me any advice. He
> says, "You are the only one who can do something about it. I
> advise you to come and sit on this throne." "I don't want to do
> that!" I exclaim. Then the lion lays his head on his front paws
> and goes to sleep. In despair I look at the other lion. He keeps
> winking at me. He says, "Why don't you do as he says. Come
> and sit here with me." When I look up again I see that the
> throne has become even higher. I take a few steps and then I
> look back to where I have come from. It doesn't feel right. From
> the height I am at I see someone approaching. It is a child. I
> bend down in order to be more or less level with her. Then we
> sit down on the throne together. The child nestles snugly against
> me. It is a big, comfortable chair. The lions are both asleep now.
>
> The throne disappears and the child and I are now sitting on
> the shore of a lake, with our feet in the water. She asks me
> whether I have made a journey. I say, "Yes, far away and high up
> and very horrible because of the pain, but it is a lot better now."

The pain that is mentioned here is not an unknown pain, occurring for the first time at this moment. What was unknown was
how it could appear so suddenly and then vanish again equally
quickly. In order to find out the answer, the Self, here represented by two lions, had to make very great demands on the ego.

In some way or other, a cramp occurred, when a great inequality in power was being experienced. At the very sight of the throne, the cramp seized hold of the body, and it was absolutely impossible for the person to mount the throne. The task was too heavy. The lion on the left smoothed the way by making the task look less awesome: "Come and sit here with me." The little girl made it possible for the woman to climb up the steps by her carefree attitude. The task was therefore stripped of all its oppressive weight.

The Self created a situation in which the imaginator was able to learn how the cramp arose and how to get rid of it, provided she was prepared to endure the trouble of such a trial.

THE PARABLE

In the imaginal world, learning takes place first of all by means of parables. The subject's own situation is compared with something else.[14] For instance, a woman going to see the Wise Man is told: "I would like you to come and watch my video." (He works with hypermodern means.)

> On the video I see a number of squares, and I run from one square to the next. One of the squares is mine, the others belong to my husband and children. My square is black from footprints.
> "How did that happen?" the Wise Man asks.
> "Well, everybody comes in through here," I say.
> He: "Why don't you guard it better then?"
> I: "I need them to come in because I am not strong enough and they come to help me."
> I: "You have plenty of strength of your own, look."
> Then I see my tree, as it was when I had raised it completely upright. Through the veins a lot of water was rising from below all the way to the top and there I was able to catch the water in cups and dole it out to the people sitting under the tree.
> He: "You see, you even have enough to share out to others. If you just let everybody enter your square you'll lose all your strength."
> "That's right," I say, "I feel dead tired and tense. I'll clean up my square first. There, that feels a lot better. Now I even have enough energy to read my book."

THE IDENTIFICATION

The parable often leads imperceptibly into an identification. You begin to compare yourself so closely with what is being presented that you become identical with it, and when that happens you can experience the events from within.

> Again I see my tree. It doesn't look too good. It has become all limp and withered. There are hardly any leaves on it anymore. The people are lying under it, gasping in the heat. They are dying from thirst. Something must be done. I am responsible for the tree and for the people and it looks as if they are all going to die. I get into the tree and feel at once what a poor state it is in. I am as limp as a dishcloth and all I want to do is flop down on the ground. This is too bad; let me first find out how my roots are doing, deep down in the earth. They feel more or less all right. Let's see if I can suck any strength up. Yes, I can. Now I can at least straighten out some of those branches up there. Look, they are getting new leaves now. That means there is a bit of shade for the people down below. The water begins to flow strongly and I can start sharing out some of it. Gradually a few smiles are returning to the faces.
>
> When I look at myself as a tree, I see there are lots of little spirals in me. I still feel as tense as a coiled spring. Let's see if I can get rid of that feeling. Yes, when I let all the cramp go, the spirals disappear. Ooh, that feels a lot better.

In identification a person does not only experience his or her own problem, but will also start looking for ways to get out of the difficulties. The image here provides a startingpoint which may lead to a satisfactory solution. The spirals turn out to be taut springs, and by loosening the tension the springs can be made to disappear from the tree. This takes us to the next point.

FEEDBACK

Before you are able to understand the images you may be unsure for a long time whether the solution that occurs to you is indeed the correct one. Sometimes you can ask someone about it, but there is not always a suitable person near by. There is nothing much you can do but try out your solution. The question which then arises is the following: by what yardstick do I measure whether my solution is right? Of course you can follow your intuition, but often you lack the necessary confidence in your own ideas. In order to strengthen this confidence the Self uses its ability to give clear feedback by means of images. These images show you whether you are going forward or backward.

In the case of the tree, above, the branches begin to stand up straight and they are acquiring new leaves. At this moment the woman does not only feel better and stronger, but she can also tell by looking at the tree that things are moving in the right direction. The image underscores the feelings.

STRUGGLING WITH THOUGHTS AND FEELINGS OF ANXIETY

A wise person in an imagination once remarked, "Anxiety does not exist, only wrong thoughts exist."

Experts will say that in this inner world all possible therapeutic approaches are utilized. As in this remark by the Wise Man, wrong thoughts lead to miserable feelings, and this is certainly true of anxiety. It is a piece of wisdom that has been known for a long time; a medicine man or shaman expresses it as follows: "Snake does not bite people; snake bites what people think."[15] Our lives can literally be made sick by the wrong kinds of thoughts and feelings. It is therefore very important that we should fight such thoughts and feelings, because if we don't, they will tyrannize our lives. At this point a difficulty often occurs, which is that in imaginations anxiety is expressed in frightening images. In their turn, these frightening images arouse anxiety. The circle is complete. It is vitally necessary to break out of this circle.

In the preceding imaginations, there have been numerous examples of such fights against the tyrants. It was for this reason that the knight and the hero played such important roles. The point is not that we should cultivate potential soldiers, but that a warrior stands up inside us, to fight the many monsters and wicked beasts in us and unmask them as phantoms of the mind.

These fights do not in fact require much violence. The monster merely needs to be told that you are not afraid of him. How this can be done we will demonstrate by a simple example.

> I see that horrid man before me again. He has witch's claws now, and he is trying to grab me by the throat with these. Now he has taken hold of me and he is squeezing my throat. How odd, he squeezes and squeezes but I do not die. I think: "Do as you like, little man." I feel my fear going away and the man shrivels up into a pathetic little creature.

That is how it is done, the horrid man was the expression of the anxiety and when the anxiety disappears the horrid man can disappear too.

Something similar happens in the following scene:

> The sky clouds over. Behind me a thunderstorm is gathering. It has become dark and the storm goes right over me. It moves very fast. All the trees in the neighborhood are hit by it. There is a terrific flash, right above my head. Behind me the water comes pouring down the street. I run as fast as I can until I reach a shed. I go inside.
>
> The door has closed behind me. I can't see any more where the storm has gone. I hear only the tremendous roar of the thunder. The flashes come right through the wooden walls. A space remains clear for me. The space around me becomes larger. The storm cannot touch me.
>
> Now I open the door because I want to see where the storm is. It seems to be losing strength. It is emptying. It doesn't have enough strength left. I watch it go, until it has completely gone.

Both these examples also demonstrate the weapon that is being used against these powers. The weapon is looking or addressing and if possible touching. You have to keep looking or start looking. In the second example the situation was at its most terrifying when the door of the shed was shut and the storm could no longer be seen. This changed when the door was opened and the person looked out to see what the enemy was like and how much strength it really had.

The fight against enemy power is not always conducted by means of force. Force may be the first means you are likely to reach for, but it is not the most effective one. You use force because you think that the opponent really has power. After a while it will become clear that this power is only apparent. As soon as you yourself begin to employ and strengthen your own power, the use of force is no longer necessary. To give an example:

> I have asked the old man to go with me into the church, because I always used to feel so miserable there. When we enter I see the Virgin Mary. She looks exactly like the statue that always stood in front of the church. Again I have those miserable feelings: I don't belong. There is no place here for me.
>
> The face of the Virgin Mary has become completely black and looks horrible. I become very angry and I want to smash her to pieces. I tell the old man so.
>
> He says, "You'd better not do that. Why don't you look whether she has something for you." Then the thought occurs to me that maybe she is having a miserable time too and that I might be able to do something for her.
>
> I go toward her and start stroking her face. Then the face becomes beautiful again. She gives me a friendly smile and says I have helped her. She gives me a flower.

For the Freedom of the Ego

As we have seen, the ego is constantly faced with choices. This is a relief in itself: the opponents and core figures do not dominate events to such an extent that the ego, as leading actor, is driven into a corner.

When we consider that in the imaginations the place of action and also many of the imaginal figures that rise up from the unconscious are often very fearsome, we realize that this freedom of the ego is not so self-evident as all that. The time for fooling around has gone, and you had better not mock the figures you meet there.

ACTING RESPONSIBLY

The time for *responsible action* has arrived. One thing we notice is
that the issuing of commands and prohibitions seems to have
been superseded. Nobody tells you what to do or not to do. You
are offered chances, you are challenged, and sometimes teased, or,
when necessary, harassed. But you are always taken seriously and
when you are unable to find your way you are offered an inex-
haustible repertoire of search programs, until you have found the
place where you have to be. All these things give you a feeling of
freedom.

You are not forced into this or that behavior, even though
sometimes you are put under fairly strong pressure. Then it almost seems as if you have lost your freedom. On some occasions it
looks as if you are being forced to be free, as in the following
example:

> I come to a large tree. Under it is a seat on which a man is sit-
> ting who has been waiting for me. He is holding a handful of
> cards, with pictures on them. He explains what the pictures
> mean and then gives the cards to me. I have to scatter them
> around me.
>
> In front of me lies a fish and that is the card he gives me.
> Then he points to the water. There is only one road I can fol-
> low. The man has suddenly vanished.
>
> The sky clouds over. It is raining. The waves become bigger
> and bigger. The path is flooded and I am now floating in the
> water. There are sounds and it is not possible to get away from
> the sounds. I don't like this. Images of myself occur, when I was
> little and afraid. I see myself as a baby. She can't sleep because of
> the noise. I can't leave her lying there. I must protect her, so I
> pick the baby up.
>
> Then I arrive in the room with the two lions. They have
> opened the door and they take the baby from me. She will be
> well looked after.

It seems as if the cards have been shuffled properly here. The
subject is not given any choice: the fish must go to the water and

there is only one way. The important point, however, is that a baby has to be rescued, which has no part in life and no freedom of choice.

The road that this woman had to take did not appeal to her at all. She had to go right through the trouble which she had always tried to avoid. Her fish lay gasping for breath on the dry land and she was compelled to take it to the water and let it swim. When she saw the situation the baby was in, her choice was clear to her. The baby could not be left to lie there.

WHO DETERMINES THE GAME?

If the freedom of choice of the main character is respected, the question still remains: who determines the game that is about to be played? Even in an extreme situation such as the one of the card game just now, the scattering of the cards is left to the woman. It is not necessary, however, to accept an enforced game. By making its wishes and desires known, the ego can often ask for a particular play-situation. If it is left open, the ego can insist that modifications are made. An example of this is the following:

> There is a very large bird overhead, an eagle. I can also see yellow sunlight and fire. It is very impressive but not frightening. The eagle wants something of me. He wants me to fly away with him, or no, more than that, he wants me to become him. Together we fly over water. I realize that I don't mind flying, but that I don't want to be that bird. I wouldn't mind having his wings, but as a woman I don't want his male body.
>
> I ask him whether something could be done just with those wings, so that I could keep my own body. He is angry now: it seems you don't ask questions like that. It can be done only if he also keeps his own body, because he doesn't want to become me either. It is getting very complicated, he says, because his body wants to go in a different direction from mine. The bird would snap apart. He says there is a possibility, but then something radical will have to be done first, when we are above land. I first want to be sure that I can keep my own body. On the beach I see a little mound of gray stuff that looks like ashes. The bird is

no longer there. I have a terrible headache, but at least I am still here.

The live drama in which you become involved in imaginations differs from the drama enacted on the stage.[16] Not only are you allowed to handle your role in any way you wish, but the actor is also free to alter the play. The relationship between the conscious and the unconscious becomes highly variable as soon as the ego enters the imaginal inner world. A strange adventure then begins, in which we can bring all our qualities to bear. You don't have to abandon your rational, analytical thought. On the contrary, it is very useful, but without intuition as well you don't get anywhere at all.

THE EGO AND THE SELF

I am surprised at my self.
I stroke my self on the head.
I begin to doubt my self.
I disregard my self.
I wish my self the best.
I don't trust my self altogether.
I run after my self.
I want to understand my self.
I am irritated by my self.
I dare not look at my self.
I am ashamed of my self.
I hide my self.
I am at odds with my self.
I let my self go.
I overestimate my self.
I flaunt my self.
I don't do justice to my self.
I could do something to my self.
I am sick of my self.
I am trapped by my self.

I want to get out of my self.
I have lost my self.
I am beside my self with rage.
I cannot forgive my self this.
I exhaust my self.
I want to get in the clear with my self.
I want to get to know my self.
I give my self courage.
I want to protect my self.
I must fight for my self.
I comfort my self.
I want to look after my self.
I can rely on my self.
I love my self.
I am my self (and so on).

NOTES

INTRODUCTION

1. Carl Gustav Jung, *Ik en Zelf,* p 10.
2. C. G. Jung, *Over grondslagen van de analytische psychologie,* p 209.
3. Richard Bandler and John Grinder, *De betovering van de taal,* p 190.

CHAPTER 1. SETTLING ACCOUNTS WITH THE PAST

1. Marie-Louise von Franz, *De vrouw in het sprookje,* p 132. (English translation: *Problems of the Feminine in Fairytales.*)
2. Friedrich W. Doucet, *Dromen en droomuitleg,* p 66.
3. Maria F. Mahoney, *De betekenis van dromen,* p 115. (English translation: *Meaning in Dreams and Dreaming.*)
4. Tom Chetwynd, *A Dictionary for Dreamers,* p 109.
5. *Herder Lexicon Symbole,* p 70.
6. F. W. Doucet, *Dromen en droomuitleg,* p 89.
7. Wolfgang Bauer, Irmtraud Dümotz, and Sergius Golowin, *Lexicon der Symbole,* p 36.

CHAPTER 2. SETTLING AN INNER CONFLICT

1. Jerome L. Singer and Kenneth S. Pope, *The Power of Imagination,* p 113.
2. R. Bandler and J. Grinder, *De betovering van de taal,* p 136.
3. Hermann Maass, *De therapeut in ons,* p 11.
4. C. G. Jung, *Ik en Zelf,* p 13.
5. Jean Chevalier and Alain Gheerbrand, *Dictionnaire des Symboles,* II p 251.

6. Mike and Nancy Samuels, *Seeing with the Mind's Eye,* p 201.

7. Emma Jung, *Animus en Anima,* p 11. (English translation: *Animus & Anima.*)

8. *Herder Lexicon Symbole,* p 73.

9. Gaston Bachelard, *The Psychoanalysis of Fire,* p 104.

10. J. E. Cirlot, *A Dictionary of Symbols,* p 322.

11. J. L. Singer and K. S. Pope, *The Power of Imagination,* p 134.

12. M. and N. Samuels, *Seeing with the Mind's Eye,* p 190.

13. Mary Anderson, *Colour Healing,* p 34.

14. J. Chevalier and A. Gheerbrand, *Dictionnaire des Symboles,* IV p 125.

15. *Herder Lexicon Symbole,* p 129.

CHAPTER 3. ANSWERS TO THE CHALLENGES OF A CIVILIZATION

1. T. Chetwynd, *A Dictionary for Dreamers,* p 52.

2. Erich Neumann, *Die Grosse Mutter.* (English translation: *The Great Mother.*)

3. M. Esther Harding, *Woman's Mysteries,* p 98.

4. Sam Keen, *The Passionate Life: Stages of Loving,* p 28.

5. *Witchcraft and Demonology,* p 219.

6. M. E. Harding, *Woman's Mysteries,* p 79.

7. J. E. Cirlot, *A Dictionary of Symbols,* p 126.

8. Nor Hall, *The Moon and the Virgin,* p 63.

9. M. E. Harding, *Woman's Mysteries,* p 230.

10. E. Neumann, *Die Grosse Mutter.* (English translation: *The Great Mother.*)

11. N. Hall, *The Moon and the Virgin,* p 109.

12. *Herder Lexicon Symbole,* p 114.

13. *Encyclopedia of World Mythology,* p 226.

14. *Herder Lexicon Symbole,* p 114.

15. N. Hall, *The Moon and the Virgin,* p 11.

16. M. E. Harding, *Woman's Mysteries,* p 193.

17. F. W. Doucet, *Dromen en droomuitleg,* p 89.

18. J. E. Cirlot, *A Dictionary of Symbols,* p 361.

19. Edward C. Whitmont, *Return of the Goddess,* p 131.

20. Mircea Eliade, *Initiaties, riten, geheime genootschappen,* p 66. (English translation: *Rites & Symbols of Initiation.*)

21. Joseph Campbell, *The Masks of God: Creative Mythology,* p 208.

22. Ibid., p 211.

23. *Encyclopedia of World Mythology,* p 122.

24. Dianne Wolkstein and Samuel Noah Kramer, *Inanna,* p 7.

CHAPTER 4. PHENOMENA AND LAWS IN THE WORLD OF THE SELF

1. Frederick S. Perls, *Gestalt Therapy Verbatim,* p 33.

2. Arnold Lazarus, *Verbeeld je beter,* p 1.

3. Claudio Naranjo and Robert E. Ornstein, *On the Psychology of Meditation,* p 216.

4. C. G. Jung, *Over grondslagen van de analytische psychologie,* p 206.

5. R. Bandler and J. Grinder, *De betovering van de taal,* p 132.

6. J. L. Singer and K. S. Pope, *The Power of Imagination,* p 132.

7. H. Maass, *De therapeut in ons,* p 11.

8. C. G. Jung, *Oerbeelden,* p 9.

9. Rüdiger Müller, *Wandlung zur Ganzheit,* p 295.

10. G. Bachelard, *The Psychoanalysis of Fire,* p vii.

12. J. L. Singer and K. S. Pope, *The Power of Imagination,* p 163.

13. R. E. Ornstein, *The Psychology of Consciousness,* p 65.

14. Bruce Joyce and Marsha Weil, *Models of Teaching,* p 238.

15. Holger Kalweit, *Traumzeit und innerer Raum,* p 7. (English translation: *Dreamtime and Inner Space.*)

16. E. C. Whitmont, *Return of the Goddess,* p 211.

BIBLIOGRAPHY

Anderson, Mary. *Colour Healing.* Wellingborough 1982.

Anderson, U. S. *The Magic in Your Mind.* Hollywood 1973.

Assagioli, Roberto. *Over de wil.* Meppel 1976. (*Act of Will.* New York 1974.)

Bachelard, Gaston. *The Psychoanalysis of Fire.* Boston 1968.

Bandler, Richard, and John Grinder. *De betovering van de taal.* Haarlem 1981.

Barz, Helmut. *Over de ziel.* Rotterdam 1981.

Bauer, Wolfgang; Irmtraud Dümotz; and Sergius Golowin. *Lexicon der Symbole.* Wiesbaden 1984.

Boenders, Frans, and Freddy Coppens. *De goden uit het Oosten.* Utrecht 1981.

Campbell, Joseph. *The Masks of God: Creative Mythology.* New York 1978.

———. *Myths to Live By.* Toronto 1982.

Chetwynd, Tom. *A Dictionary for Dreamers.* London 1972.

Chevalier, Jean, and Alain Gheerbrand. *Dictionnaire des Symboles.* Paris 1974.

Cirlot, J. E. *A Dictionary of Symbols.* New York 1983.

Colegrave, Sukie. *Androgynie.* Rotterdam 1981.

Dieckmann, Hans. *Omgaan met dromen.* Rotterdam 1981. (*Twice-Told Tales: The Psychological Use of Fairy Tales.* Boris Matthews, trans. from Ger. Wilmett, I. L. 1986.)

Doucet, Friedrich W. *Dromen en droomuitleg.* Delft.

Dürkheim, Karlfried Graf von. *Transcendentaal ervaren.* Katwijk 1980.

———. *De roep om een meester.* Katwijk 1982. (*The Call for the Master: The Meaning of Spiritual Leadership on the Way to the Self.* De Angelis, Paul, ed., Nash, Vincent, tr. New York 1989.)

———. *Die zielfreie Weg.* Freiburg 1982. (*Way of Transformation.* Winchester, M.A. 1980.)

Eliade, Mircea. *Shamanismus und archaische Ekstasetechnik.* Frankfurt

1975. (*Shamanism: Archaic Techniques of Ecstasy*, trans. Willard R. Trask. Bollingen Ser.:Vol 76. Princeton, N.J. 1964.)

———. *Initiaties, riten, geheime genootschappen.* Katwijk 1984. (*Rites and Symbols of Initiation: The Mysteries of Birth & Rebirth.* [Original title: *Birth & Rebirth*] New York 1958.)

Eliot, Alexander. *Mythen van de mensheid.* Amsterdam 1977.

Encyclopedia of World Mythology. London 1975.

Encyclopedia of Magic and Superstition. London 1974.

Faure, Paul. *Kreta.* Stuttgart 1978.

Ferguson, Marilyn. *De aquarius Samenzwering.* Deventer 1983. (*The Aquarian Conspiracy: Personal and Social Transformation in the 1980s.* Los Angeles 1981 [rev. ed. 1987].)

Fromm, Erich. *Dromen, sprookjes, mythen,* Utrecht 1980.

Garfield, Patricia. *Creatief dromen.* Utrecht 1980. (*Creative Dreaming.* New York 1976.)

Halifax, Joan. *Die andere Wirklichkeit der Schamanen.* Bern 1983. (*Shamanic Voices: A Survey of Visionary Narratives.* Dutton 1979.)

Hall, Nor. *The Moon and the Virgin.* New York 1960.

Hamilton, Edith. *Mythology.* New York 1969.

Harding, M. Esther. *Woman's Mysteries.* London 1971.

Harner, Michael. *Der Weg der Schamanen.* Interlaken 1983. (*The Way of the Shaman.* New York 1982.)

Herder Lexicon Symbole. Freiburg 1978.

Hillman, James. *Am Anfang war das Bild.* München 1982.

Jacobi, Jolande. *Vom Bilderreich der Seele.* Olten 1981. (*The Way of Individuation.* New York 1983.)

Jahoda, Gustav. *The Psychology of Superstition.* Harmondsworth 1970.

Jones, Richard M. *Fantasy and Feeling in Education.* Harmondsworth 1972.

Joyce, Bruce, and Marsha Weil. *Models of Teaching.* Englewood Cliffs, N.J. 1972.

Jung, Carl Gustav. *Herinneringen dromen gedachten.* Rotterdam 1978. (*Memories, Dreams, Reflections,* ed. Aniela Jaffé; trans. Richard Winston and Clara Winston. New York 1963.)

———. *Over grondslagen van de analytische psychologie.* Rotterdam 1978.

———. *Archetypen.* Katwijk 1981.

———. *Ik en zelf.* Rotterdam 1982.

———. *Oerbeelden.* Rotterdam 1982.

————. *De mens en zijn symbolen.* Rotterdam 1985. (*Man and His Symbols,* with Marie-Louise von Franz, J. L. Henderson, Jolande Jacobi, and Aniela Jaffé. New York 1969. Reproduction of the 1964 edition.)

Jung, Emma. *Animus en anima.* Rotterdam 1983. (*Animus and Anima.* Dallas 1985.)

Kalweit, Holger. *Traumzeit und innerer Raum.* Bern 1984. (*Dreamtime and Inner Space: The World of the Shaman.* Boston & London, 1988.)

Keen, Sam. *The Passionate Life: Stages of Loving.* San Francisco 1983.

Kopp, Sheldon B. *De psychotherapie als pelgrimstocht.* Utrecht 1981.

Larousse New Encyclopedia of Mythology. London 1978.

Latner, Joel. *The Gestalt Therapy Book.* New York 1974.

Lazarus, Arnold. *Verbeeld je beter.* Lisse 1980.

Lindenberg, Vladimir. *Riten und Stufen der Einweihung.* Freiburg 1978.

Maass, Hermann. *De therapeut in ons.* Rotterdam 1982.

Mahoney, Maria F. *De beteknis van dromen.* Rotterdam 1982. (*Meaning in Dreams and Dreaming.* Lyle Stuart 1966.)

Marcuse, Herbert. *Eros en cultuur.* Utrecht 1971. (*Eros and Civilization: A Philosophical Inquiry into Freud.* Boston 1974.)

Moody, Raymond A. *Leven na dit leven.* Bussum 1978. (*Life after Life.* New York 1984.)

Müller, Rüdiger. *Wandlung zur Ganzheit.* Freiburg 1981.

Naranjo, Claudio, and Robert E. Ornstein. *On the Psychology of Meditation.* New York, 1973.

Neumann, Erich. *Die grosse Mutter.* Olten 1981. (*The Great Mother: An Analysis of the Archetype,* trans. Ralph Manheim. Princeton, N.J. 1964.)

Ornstein, Robert E. *The Psychology of Consciousness.* Harmondsworth 1981.

Pavitt, William. *Het boek der talismans, amuletten en zodiakale stenen.* Amsterdam 1979. (*Book of Talismans, Amulets, and Zodiacal Gems.* London 1929)

Perls, Frederick S. *Gestalt Therapy Verbatim.* New York 1972.

Riemann, Fritz. *Psychologie van de angst.* 's-Gravenhage 1980.

Romé, Jesús. *The Civilization of the Maya.* Geneva 1979.

Samuels, Mike and Nancy. *Seeing with the Mind's Eye.* New York 1983.

Sanford, John A. *De onbekende partner.* Rotterdam 1982. (*Invisible Partners.* New Jersey 1980.)

Schmidbauer, W. *Van magie tot psychotherapie.* Haarlem 1973.

Schutz, Will, and Evelyn Turner. *Body Fantasy.* New York 1977, 1985.

184   BIBLIOGRAPHY

Singer, Jerome L., and Kenneth S. Pope. *The Power of Imagination.* New York 1978.
Stanislawsky, Konstantin S. *Theater, Regie und Schauspieler.* Hamburg 1958.
Storr, Anthony. *Jung: Selected Writings.* London 1983.
von Franz, Marie-Louise. *De vrouw in het sprookje.* Rotterdam 1980. (*Problems of the Feminine in Fairytales.* Dallas 1972.)
———. *De werkelijkheid in het sprookje,* Rotterdam 1981.
Whitmont, Edward C. *Return of the Goddess.* London 1983.
Witchcraft and Demonology. London 1974.
Wolkstein, Dianne, and Samuel Noah Kramer. *Inanna.* New York 1983.
Wunderlich, H. G. *The Secret of Crete.* London 1975.

9 781570 627002